Overthinking:

27 Most Powerful Steps to Stop Overthinking and Declutter Your Mind! Achieve Spiritual Mindfulness with Daily Meditation and Create Successful Habits for Successful Life!

© **Copyright by Tony Bennis 2019 - All rights reserved.**

The content contained within this book may not be reproduced, duplicated or transmitted without direct written permission from the author or the publisher.

Under no circumstances will any blame or legal responsibility be held against the publisher, or author, for any damages, reparation, or monetary loss due to the information contained within this book. Either directly or indirectly.

Legal Notice:

This book is copyright protected. This book is only for personal use. You cannot amend, distribute, sell, use, quote or paraphrase any part, or the content within this book, without the consent of the author or publisher.

Disclaimer Notice:

Please note the information contained within this document is for educational and entertainment purposes only. All effort has been executed to present accurate, up to date, and reliable, complete information. No warranties of any kind are declared or implied. Readers acknowledge that the author is not engaging in the rendering of legal, financial, medical or professional advice. The content within this book has been derived from various sources. Please consult a licensed professional before attempting any techniques outlined in this book.

By reading this document, the reader agrees that under no circumstances is the author responsible for any losses, direct or indirect, which are incurred as a result of the use of information contained within this document, including, but not limited to, — errors, omissions, or inaccuracies.

Table of Contents

Introduction..................8

Chapter 1: What is Overthinking? 10

    Why Do We Overthink?

    The Overthinking Brain

    Overthinking Symptoms

    Dangers of Being an Over-Thinker

    Three Types of Overthinking

Chapter 2: Anxiety and Overthinking..................20

    Ways Anxiety Causes Overthinking

    Result of Anxiety and Overthinking

    What Overthinking Is Not

    How to Stop Overthinking Everything

Chapter 3: Try to Stop it Before it Starts..................26

    Limiting Beliefs

    Unhelpful Coping Strategies

    Prepare to Train Your Brain To Establish A Healthy Relationship With Your Thoughts

Chapter 4: Focus on Active Problem-Solving..................32

    What Is Active Problem-Solving?

    Questions To Ask Yourself

When Is Active Problem-Solving Effective?

How to Use Active Problem-Solving

Chapter 5: Consider the Worst-Case Scenario..................38

What to Do When Considering The Worst-Case Scenario

Why You Should Consider the Worst-Case Scenario

Chapter 6: Schedule Thinking Time..................43

The "Schedule Thinking Time " Steps.

Chapter 7: Think Usefully..................48

Chapter 8: Set Time Limits for Making Decisions..................53

How to Set Time Limits For Your Decisions

Set A Limit To The Number Of Decisions You Make Per Day.

Chapter 9: Consider the Bigger Picture..................58

Chapter 10: Live in the Moment..................64

Why Is It Important To Be Present?

Practical Steps To Living In The Present.

Chapter 11: Meditate..................69

4 Ways in Which Meditation Helps To Stop Overthinking

How to Meditate In 9 Simple Steps

Chapter 12: Create A To-Do List..................75

Chapter 13: Embrace Positivity..................81

Chapter 14: Using Affirmations to Harness Positive Thinking.................86

    What Are Affirmations And Do They Work?

    How to Use Positive Affirmations

    How to Write an Affirmation Statement

    Examples of Affirmations

Chapter 15: Become Action-Oriented.................93

    Tips to Taking Action in Overcoming Overthinking

Chapter 16: Overcoming Your Fear.................97

Chapter 17: Trust Yourself.................100

Chapter 18: Stop Waiting for the Perfect Moment.................106

Chapter 19: Stop Setting your Day up for Stress and Overthinking.................111

Chapter 20: Accepting Everything that Happens.................114

    Ways to Let Go of Past Hurts

Chapter 21: Give Your Best and Forget the Rest.................120

    It Doesn't Have To Be Difficult.

Chapter 22: Don't put Pressure on Yourself to Handle it.................125

Chapter 23: Journal to get the Thoughts out of your Head.................129

    How to Get Started

    Journaling Your Way to a Better Frame Of Mind

Chapter 24: Change the Channel.................133

Chapter 25: Take A Break.................136

   Break for Results

Chapter 26: Work out.................140

   How Exercise Promotes Positive Well-Being

   Types of Exercises to Overcome Overthinking

Chapter 27: Get a Hobby.................145

Chapter 28: Don't Be Too Hard On Yourself.................148

   How to Stop Being Too Hard on Yourself

Chapter 29: Get Plenty of Good Quality Sleep.................152

   Benefits of Sleeping

   How to Get The Most From Your Sleep

Conclusion.................159

References.................161

Introduction

Overthinking is very common and debilitating. It can hinder you from socializing, from having a sound sleep, affect your performance at work, and even disrupt a well-planned vacation. When overthinking becomes chronic, it can lead to both physical and mental discomfort. In summary, overthinking can leave you both physically and mentally exhausted. If this is how you feel at the moment, you might have attempted various ways of escaping from such a depressing situation with no success.

But then, what is overthinking disorder? Under normal circumstances, we all worry about one thing or another but when such anxieties begin to suck the life out of us, then it becomes a serious problem. Although not everyone will suffer from such degree of worries, some individuals are more prone to suffer from such disorders than others - especially people with a past record of anxiety disorder. Scientists have discovered that overthinking can activate various areas of the brain that regulate anxiety and fear.

But even if you never had a history of anxiety disorder, you might still be prone to overthinking, especially if you assume the responsibility of being a "problem-solver". Your greatest strength as an analytical thinker can end up becoming your greatest enemy, especially when you get stuck in a quagmire of unproductive thoughts. Also, feelings of uncertainty to a high degree can induce overthinking disorder. For instance, if a significant change such as a major loss occurred in your life, you might lose control of your mind and it may spin in an unproductive obsessiveness direction.

It is comforting to learn that one can overcome overthinking (and anxiety). There are many effective techniques for solving anxieties, no matter the cause, be it overthinking due to a failed relationship, health, or financial issues. Stay tuned, as this book takes you through the techniques of how to stop overthinking. But first, this book will start by defining each problem and then discussing the most effective solutions for each problem.

Chapter 1: What is Overthinking?

As the name implies, overthinking simply means thinking too much. In reality, when you spend more time thinking instead of acting and engaging in other activities, then you're overthinking. You can find yourself analyzing, commenting, and repeating the same thoughts over and over again, rather than taking action, then you're overthinking. Such bad habits can hinder your progress, leaving one unproductive.

Each individual will experience overthinking differently and no two people overthink the same way. But generally, all those who overthink will agree that the quality of their life has been affected by their inability to control their negative thoughts and emotions. Such habits make it very difficult for the majority of the individuals to socialize, be productive at work, or enjoy hobbies due to the enormous amount of time and energy their mind consumes on a specific line of thoughts. Such uncontrolled emotions can be very harmful to the individual's mental health.

Overthinking makes it more difficult to make new friends and to keep friends, you will find it difficult to converse with them because you're overly concerned about what to say or what to do to keep the conversation going. Some individuals who are affected by this disorder may find it challenging to participate in general conversations or to interact with others even in a normal environment. In addition, some may have trouble keeping an appointment or going to the store. This kind of thinking wastes time and drains your energy, thereby preventing you from taking action or exploring new ideas. It also hinders progress in life. This can be compared to attaching a chain that is connected to a pole around your waist and then running in circles you will be busy but not productive. Overthinking will disable your capacity to make sound decisions.

Under such circumstances, you're more likely to be worried, anxious, and devoid of inner peace of mind. However, when you stop overthinking, you will become more productive, happy, and will enjoy more peace.

Why Do We Overthink?

So far, there are two major explanations for the reason people overthink:

- The overthinking brain and
- Contemporary culture.

The Overthinking Brain

Our brain is designed in such a way that all our thoughts are interconnected in networks and nodes. For instance, thoughts about work may be in one network, and thoughts about family in another.

There is a strong connection between our emotions and moods. Activities or circumstances that stimulate negative feelings seem to be connected to one network, while those that induce happiness are linked to another network.

Although such interconnectedness of feeling and thought can help people to think more efficiently, it can also make people overthink.

In general, negative moods often activate negative thoughts and memories, even if such thoughts are unrelated. Overthinking while in a negative mood can fill the mind with lots of negative ideas and the more such a person overthinks, the easier it will be for his brain to induce negative associations.

According to research by brain experts, it has been discovered that damage (or miswiring) of certain areas of the brain can make one prone to depression and overthinking. Such areas include the amygdala and hippocampus, which are involved in learning and remembering, and the prefrontal cortex, which helps to regulate emotions. This knowledge partly explains why some individuals overthink more than others.

The Overthinking Generation. The reports from the studies conducted by the author showed that young ones, as well as middle-aged individuals, do overthink even more than the elderly ones (those above 65 years) do.

What can be responsible for this? There are 4 possible cultural trends that can be responsible:

- **Entitlement obsession:** Many today have an overdeveloped sense of entitlement. They are entitled to be rich, successful, and happy and as such, no one can hinder them from getting what they deserve. Thus, most people worry because they aren't getting what they deserve, they try to find out what is holding them back. Such overthinking attitude has turned many into a ticking bomb, ready to explode at the slightest provocation.

- **The vacuum of values:** Majority of people today, especially the youth, have questioned all the values their parents handed over to them such as religion, culture, and social norms. Therefore, such ones are left with only a few choices and without values, such a person will end up questioning each choice he makes and keep wondering if he made the right choice. (This too can lead overthinking).

- **Belly button culture:** Modern culture and popular psychology often encourage people to be more expressive and to develop more self-awareness. However, most people often take this to the extreme, thereby becoming excessively self-absorbed, they overanalyze themselves and their feelings. Many people waste too much time "staring at their navels," brainstorming over the meaning of each emotional change.

- **The compulsive need for quick fixes:** The 21st century is filled with people who tend to search for quick fixes, instead of taking time to gradually work things out. For instance, if someone is sad or troubled, he can resort to some quick way out such as drinking alcohol, shopping, taking prescription drugs, engaging in a new sport or hobby, or some other activities. In summary, quick fixes only provide a temporary solution (or even wrong solution).

Overthinking Symptoms

Having a well-defined list of overthinking symptoms can be quite helpful. In fact, awareness is your best defense, it will help you to know when you are in the danger zone, and failure to be on guard is very dangerous for your mental well-being.

Watching out for the following symptoms can help you carry out an overthinking disorder test. If you observe that you are experiencing the overthinking disorder, you may observe one or more of these following symptoms:

- **When you can't sleep:** Try as hard as you may to get a decent rest, but your mind won't just turn off.

Then agitation and worries sets in.

- **If you self-medicate:** Research on overthinking disorder has shown that those suffering from it often resort to food, alcohol, drugs, or any means of modulating feelings.

- **You're usually tired:** Tiredness can be as a result of insomnia, or due to repeated thinking which drains the strength out of you.

- **You want to be in control everything:** You attempt to plan all aspects of your life to the very last detail. But the truth is, there's a limit to what you can control.

- **You obsess about failure:** The fear of failure has made you turn into a perfectionist and you often imagine how bad things will turn out if things don't work out well.

- **You fear the future**: Rather than being thrilled by what the future holds, you're stuck in your thoughts.

- **You doubt your own judgment:** You reconsider every decision you make from what you wear, to what you say, and how you relate with others.

- **You get tension headaches:** You might experience chronic tension headaches as though a tight band is around your temples. In addition, you might also feel pain or stiffness around the neck region. All these are signs that you need a long rest.

If any of the above signs happen all too often, psychologists will say you're an over-thinker or a ruminator. According to psychologists, over-thinking can affect performance, cause anxiety, or even lead to depression.

Dangers of Being an Over-Thinker

If you still feel bad about a mistake you made weeks ago or you're anxious about tomorrow, the fact is, overthinking everything can affect your health negatively. Being unable to break free from your worries will lead you into a state of persistent anguish.

It is true that we all overthink situations occasionally. But this is different from being a true over-thinker, someone who struggles to silence his constant barrages of thoughts.

Three dangers of being an over-thinker:

1. **It increases your chances of mental illness:** According to a 2013 study which was published in the Journal of Abnormal Psychology, the reports show that overthinking about your mistakes, shortcomings, and challenges can increase your risk of mental health illness.

    Rumination is detrimental to mental health and can plunge one into a vicious cycle that is hard to break free from and as your mental health nose-dives, you tend to ruminate more.

2. **It interferes with problem-solving.** Reports

from various researchers have shown that over-thinkers always assume that by rehashing their problems in their heads, they're helping themselves. But this isn't true at all, rather, many studies showed that such actions can lead to analysis paralysis.

When we overanalyze everything, it can interfere with our ability to solve our problems. You will end up wasting time thinking about the problem rather than on the possible solution.

It will also affect the simple decision-making process such as choosing what to wear to Thanksgiving or deciding when to go on vacation. The painful part is that overthinking won't even aid you in making a better choice.

3. **It affects your sleep:** As an over-thinker, you will likely understanding this fact quite well. Anytime your mind refuses to shut off, then there will be no sleep that night.

   Studies support this fact, and there is evidence that anxiety and rumination will lead to fewer hours of sleep. You are more likely to spend hours rolling up and down the bed before you finally drift off.

   Taking a nap, later on, may not be of any help, anxiety and overthinking affects the quality sleep you will get, the chances of falling into a deep slumber after you've been thinking is very slim.

Three Types of Overthinking

1. Rant-and-rave overthinking: This is the most common type and it often results from some perceived wrongdoing which was done to you. You may feel you were unjustly treated and, as such, you're overly obsessed about taking revenge. Though you may be right by feeling offended, overthinking will prevent you from seeing the good in others, rather, you will only see them as villains. Such feelings can result in self-destructive and impulsive acts of revenge. For instance, when rejected at a job interview, an over-thinker can begin to think of the evaluators as biased or stupid and can even consider suing the company for possible discrimination.

2. Life-of-their-own overthinking: This too is another serious problem of over-thinkers. A simple stimulus can lead to a continuous cycle of vicious negative thoughts and endless possibilities, each more evil than the previous one. Take, for example, an over-thinker who begin to wonder why he feels depressed and from there, he moves on to thinking about being overweight, why he shouldn't keep close friends, why he is being treated badly at work, and why he is being unloved at home. To him, all these negative feelings appear true, even imaginary thoughts. Such negative feelings can lead to bad decisions, such as quarreling with his wife or friends or even quitting his job.

3. Chaotic overthinking: This is a kind of overthinking that is characterized by random, unrelated worries and concerns. This can be mentally and emotionally paralyzing because these ones are confused about the real cause of how they are feeling. Most often, such individuals resort to drugs or alcohol abuse, just to escape from their thoughts.

Chapter 2: Anxiety and Overthinking.

One of the terrifying signs of any form of anxiety disorder is the propensity to overthink everything. Anxiety and overthinking can be called evil partners. An anxious brain is always hypervigilant and on the watch for any possible danger. Probably someone has once accused you of always creating problems for yourself out of insignificant issues. Personally, I think they are actually problems. How so? Simply put, anxiety makes you overthink anything and everything. Whenever we are anxious, we overthink things in various ways, and the product of our overthinking is not often beneficial. However, anxiety and overthinking should be temporary and should not be a permanent feature of our existence.

Ways Anxiety Causes Overthinking

The end product of various types of anxiety is overthinking everything. There are various terms to describe how anxiety leads to overthinking. It is possible that this generic list will help you recall specific racing thoughts which you may have experienced or are likely experiencing and thus, help you realize that there are thousands of other individuals facing the same problem.

- Being overly concerned about who we are and how others view us or if we are measuring up to the world standard (this is a form of social and performance anxiety).

- Obsessing over what we should say/said/should have said/shouldn't say (another common social anxiety).

- Thinking about fearful possible scenarios such as: what if something bad should happen to us, our loved ones, or even the world (a common form of generalized anxiety disorder).

- Fearful, assumed results of our own wild thoughts, assumed faults, and feelings of incompetence (all forms of anxiety disorders).

- Anxiety over multiple obsessive thoughts, mostly scary ones, and thinking about them continually (a form of obsessive, compulsive disorder).

- Thinking, overthinking, vague thoughts, a tumbling chain of anxiety, and specific thoughts (all forms of anxiety disorders).

- Fear of experiencing panic attacks in public and feeling too scared to leave home due to such anxiety (a form of panic disorder with/without agoraphobia).

Result of Anxiety and Overthinking

When you're anxious, the thoughts do not just run through your brain and disappear, rather, they run through your brain continuously. Those thoughts can be compared to an athlete running on a treadmill, he keeps running but gets nowhere in the end, left wired and tired. One of the side effects of overthinking linked with anxiety is that we are likely to end up both physically and emotionally drained. Having bouts of the same anxious impulses run through our brain will definitely take its toll.

Another dark side of anxiety and overthinking is that sooner or later, we will begin to perceive everything that goes through our mind as reality. Perhaps we may believe that what we think about becomes reality and if we constantly think about it, it becomes very real. Right? No. This is one of the tricks anxiety tries to play on our minds.

But the good news is, we all have the capacity and the power to stop ourselves from being anxious and overthinking everything. Although, this is a process that involves multiple steps, at the moment, the best step you can take is to find something that can distract you from overthinking. Instead of battling with your thoughts, lowly divert your attention to something neutral, something else entirely. By pondering over something that is of no significance, you will be indirectly preventing overthinking everything.

The "leaven" effect

Overthinking has a "leaven effect" on your thoughts. Just like a dough, your mind can knead negative thoughts and, before you know it, it will rise to twice the initial size. For instance, if a customer is dissatisfied with your services, you may begin to wonder if all the other customers are dissatisfied as well without giving it a second thought that probably most of the customers might actually be satisfied with your services. If care is not taken, with time, you might come to a discouraging conclusion that your services are not good enough. Your thoughts can even take you back to your marriage and you might begin to wonder if your mate is satisfied with you or if you're good enough for her or not. You think about how perfect she is, how she handles everything impressively, and conclude that you're totally unworthy of her.

The "distorted lens" effect

Another effect of overthinking is what is called the "distorted lens" effect and what this means, is that your thoughts only focus and magnify your faults or bad side and what your thoughts see is only hopelessness. For instance, when your kid comes home from school with a poor grade or gets into a fight, you may worry that he or she is growing up badly. Before long, you will start seeing yourself as a bad parent and that later in the future, your children will end up becoming bad adults.

What Overthinking Is Not

Worrying is quite different from overthinking. People often worry about things that can or may happen or possibly go wrong. Overthinkers; however, do more than just worry about the present, they also worry about the past and the future as well. While worriers think that bad things might happen; over thinkers think backward and they are very convinced that something bad had already happened.

Individuals with obsessive-compulsive disorder (OCD) are also different from overthinking. Those with OCD are overly obsessed about everything or every external factor, such as dirt or germs so they feel they have to wash their hands repeatedly to stay healthy. Such ones obsess about very specific actions and other matters that appear trivial or absurd to the rest of the world, such as "Did I lock the door?"

Conclusively, overthinking is definitely not "deep thinking." While it is healthy to be in tune with one's feelings in order to examine one's actions; overthinking, on the other hand, is unhealthy.

How to Stop Overthinking Everything

Whether you've not bought a new car in the past 5 years because you haven't found that perfect one or you've not been productive because each choice you make consumes so much time, overthinking can delay your progress.

Gladly, you can overcome overthinking and become more productive. In the next 27 chapters, there are different steps that have been broken down to help you stop overthinking everything. By applying new techniques and learning new skills, you will be able to make good and timely choices with little or no stress.

Chapter 3: Try to Stop it Before it Starts.

Be in charge of your thoughts before you jump into the dark pit of overthinking, it is imperative for you to first clarify what you're actually overthinking about and also reflect on the negative ways overthinking is affecting your life. Such clarity will help enhance your determination to fight the tendency of overthinking.

Limiting Beliefs

The first thing you need to do is to pick out the "what if" questions you might likely ask yourself. Such questions are automatically stimulants of overthinking.

Ask yourself:

- What are the common "what if" questions that I usually ask myself?
- What circumstances or situations often trigger these questions?

It can be that you're overthinking because you often ask the wrong questions. Most often, rather than seeking solutions to the problem, you're busy painting "what if" scenarios in your mind, wondering about all the possible negative things that can occur.

So, take a deep breath and try to identify all the "what if" questions you often ask yourself. Also, try to detect specific circumstances that are likely to trigger such questions.

The next step is to dig into any limiting beliefs you might have, and try to gain a better understanding of some of the effect such thoughts have on your worries.

Ask yourself:

- What are my "thoughts" about overthinking?
- How do such beliefs affect the choices and decisions I make?
- Do such thoughts have any advantages?
- What are the long-term side effects of such beliefs?

When you are overthinking something, it is clear evidence that you're holding onto a certain set of beliefs which is affecting how you think and how you respond in such a situation. To face the fact, you're holding on to such beliefs because you feel they are of advantage to you. Probably, you feel they are advantageous because they give you a sense of control over certain circumstances or specific areas of your life. But sadly, such beliefs are hurting you because they hinder you from dealing with the major reasons why you're overthinking and that is a serious problem itself.

The best way to conquer your limiting beliefs is to

challenge them head-on. Listed below are a few examples of certain questions you can ask yourself:

- Why do I believe that I can't control overthinking?
- Why do I believe that overthinking is beneficial?
- Is there any evidence to back such thoughts?
- Is the evidence credible and reliable?
- Is it possible for me to view this situation from another angle?
- Do I have any evidence that goes against my beliefs about this?
- What do these tell me about my bad habit of overthinking?

If you dedicate more time to diligently questioning your limiting beliefs about overthinking, you will discover that such deep thinking is beneficial, as you will detect more holes and all these will make it easy for you to abandon such beliefs and therefore, strengthen your determination to keep searching for solutions to your problems.

All the thoughts that lead to overthinking are simply problems that you need to solve. But, if you're constantly swimming in a pool of uncontrollable worries, you will never be able to solve your problems.

Unhelpful Coping Strategies

At this point, take a moment to reflect on some of the strategies you regularly use to cope with your thoughts then,

Ask yourself:

- What are the strategies I employ to cope with my thoughts?
- What do I do to avoid my worries?
- What are some strategies that I have tried to control my thoughts?
- Do I usually suppress my thoughts? If yes, how?
- Do I often attempt to distract myself from my worries? If so, in what specific ways?
- How do I usually handle my worries?
- In what specific ways do all these coping strategies help me?
- How do these coping strategies hurt me?
- What are some better ways to manage my worries?

Gaining such clarity about the common strategies which you regularly use to manage your worries will help you get some valuable feedback which you can effectively use to control your worries in the future.

Prepare to Train Your Brain To Establish A Healthy Relationship With Your Thoughts

Your thoughts are definitely different from reality. However, your thoughts can have a strong impact on you in real life, depending on how you view them.

Discard the saying that you're your thoughts. Rather, seek for ways to establish a connection with your thoughts and to maintain a healthy relationship with it.

If you observe that a particular thought keeps popping up in your mind, you can ask yourself these questions:

- Do I perceive this thought as just a mental construct or I believe it to be the reality?

- Do such thoughts keep me up all night, or do I just let them go?

- Do I accept the thoughts just the way they come or attempt to change them?

- Am I open to other thoughts or do I simply shut myself away from them?

- What thoughts does this thought awaken in me?

After posing such questions, wait for the answers to come up— though the answers may not be obvious at first, posing such questions is very important. Gradually, you will be able to relate to your thoughts.

You can simply ask, "But is this true?"

The best kind of relationship you can establish with your thoughts is one that is full of acceptance and yet a measure of healthy distance. What this means is that you're open to any thoughts and you don't try to act as though they don't exist; however, you can also try as much as possible not to let them pull you down.

For instance, if you had a bad experience with a lousy cashier, you can begin to think that things might actually be better if only you had gone to another check-out, but you don't need to believe such mental interpretations because they are mere assumptions and not the ultimate reality. What are the possibilities? Probably this particular person is a wonderful cashier who is just having a bad day and maybe if you chose the other line you will still be on the queue. Such thoughts keep you open to possibilities.

When you compliment yourself or you acknowledge that you feel like you did well, you tend to enjoy such feelings. For instance, when you tell yourself: "Well done me! I led the team all the way to the top!" However, this doesn't mean your performance in the next game will be the same. It also doesn't make you a "better person" because your self-worth is not attached to how well you can lead a team.

Always challenge your thoughts. Learn to identify and stop any extra thoughts.

Chapter 4: Focus on Active Problem-Solving.

Active ways of solving problems are one of the most valuable skills that we need but we rarely think about in our busy daily lives. Rather, we often focus our attention on trying to tackle the various difficult emotions we face. It is true that we also need coping skills in order to limit overthinking, but it is equally important for us to arm ourselves with skills we can use to manage or cope with problems that cause overthinking. This is the role that active problem-solving skills play.

We need to understand that there are certain circumstances that are beyond our power and which we can't change. Thus, overthinking about such types of circumstances is of no benefit. However, you don't have to stop looking for ways to solve other problems simply because you can't see an obvious solution.

We need to understand the difference between productive problem-solving skills and overthinking. Some of the characteristics of overthinking include the following:

- It makes you repeat the same thoughts over and over.
- It makes you keep seeking "solutions" to problems you know you don't have the power to change.

- It makes you focus your attention on changing things that already happened in the past.

However, problem-solving skills have the following characteristics:

- It doesn't make you think about the same thing over and over again.

- It ends up producing alternative solutions, most of which are within your capacity to execute.

- It makes you feel positive, and feel like you're accomplishing something worthwhile even before a solution is reached.

What Is Active Problem-Solving?

It is often more effective and beneficial to focus on trying to solve the problem at hand than trying to control how you feel about the problem. Facing your problems head-on will help you gain control of your life with less stress. This process of handling problems is known as active problem-solving. It focuses on making active efforts to solve the problem from the root, rather than overlooking the problem.

However, this processing is not as easy as it sounds. Facing our problems directly can be very difficult at times. This is because you have to confront your fears, approach conflicts, or at times, move out of your comfort zone until the problem is resolved. But active problem-solving actually has long term benefits because it helps to reduce future discomfort since the problem is no longer disturbing your mind.

Questions To Ask Yourself

There are various reasons why you need to ask yourself these questions. It can be that you have doubts about the business moves you plan to take, or you are facing some challenges in your relationship, finding answers to these questions will help you to know whether you're the overthinking or problem-solving type.

- **Do I always focus on the problem or do I search for a solution?** Considering various ways of getting out of debt can be helpful. But focusing your attention or worrying about what will happen if you eventually become homeless due to your financial condition is not the way forward.

- **Is there a solution to this problem?** It is good to accept the fact that not all problems can be solved. For instance, a loved one with a terminal disease, or a mistake which you already made in the past can't be undone. However, you can still control how you respond to such situations. Problem-solving can involve learning to heal your emotions or an actual solving the problem procedure. But overthinking, on the other hand, involves rehashing things that already happened or wishing things were different.

- **What will I accomplish by thinking about this?** Assuming you're going through a past event to gain new insight or learn from it, this might be helpful. But if all you're doing is replaying your mistakes, rehashing a past conversation, or just imagining all the things that can possibly go wrong, then you're overthinking.

When Is Active Problem-Solving Effective?

In life, there are some situations we cannot control. In this kind of situation, no active problem-solving plan can change things. All we have to do is endure and then move on.

You can't solve a problem you don't have control over. Most of these problems have to do with the decisions of other people. For instance, your sister has just made a decision to get married to her long-time lover and you, on the other hand, are against the decision. Now, the decision is not yours to make, so you cannot control the situation. Therefore, you cannot solve it.

Looking at another scenario, where the heat in your house is not functioning and that has caused a problem between you and your landlord. This situation can either be solved by an active-problem-solving because it is under your control or you can decide to endure the cold house using emotion-focused skills.

How to Use Active Problem-Solving

Evaluate the situation Certain things affect us daily; some people dwell on them so much that it steals their joy and happiness. When we encounter issues like these, we should first of all evaluate the situation. Before handling any problem, you will have to assess the problem at hand. Consider whether you can control the outcome of events, if the problem can be solved or endured. If it can be solved, how can you go about it? All these taken into consideration will help you handle situations or problems better.

Determine the most effective course of action. After the first stage, where you evaluate the situation and you realize that it can be solved. The next stage is choosing the most appropriate measure for tackling the problem.

Taking the illustration of the landlord and tenant problem stated above, there are different ways to solve that problem. One way to go about it is yelling at the landlord and making sure that his life is a living hell until he gets the heat fixed. The other option can be writing a letter to your landlord, explaining the problem you are facing with the heat, then you document a copy for yourself. However, this should be done based on the tenant's right in your province. Now, there are two options that can fix the problem but which is the most appropriate?

The first option may seem easier and faster but think about the consequences. No landlord will be happy with such reaction and this may create more problems for you. However, the latter is the most effective course of action.

It can be hard to make decisions alone, especially when emotion is involved. Therefore, seek the counsel of good friends or therapists who can help you to see better options.

Turn overthinking into problem-solving. What's the need of overthinking when you can solve the problem? Overthinking does you no good, rather it consumes the energy you will have used to solve the problem and achieve a purpose. Be very conscious to stop yourself whenever you are forced to overthink. Therefore, instead of wasting your time and energy to worry, use it for active problem-solving. This will not just give you peace of mind, but you will be able to get rid of some problems.

Know the difference between problem-solving and worrying.

Chapter 5: Consider the Worst-Case Scenario.

It seems a bit impractical, right? When you are totally scared and overburdened by stress, one thing you will not want to do is to think about the worst possible scenario. Right?

Our mind tells us convincing stories. Our thoughts are powerful enough to decide what we do or do not do. One method of controlling overthinking is to imagine the worst possible scenario.

If you are overthinking, there will be an increase in your mental effort and this will negatively influence your performance. Making plans for a difficult situation ensures that you are prepared for any horrible feeling during the course of the event, so you are preparing yourself to maximize all your potential.

To redirect your thoughts into more positive ones, here are three short personal affirmations. By using one or more of them, you can achieve calmness and continue.

"It is not happening presently." Sure, it is definitely likely that an unfortunate event might happen, but it is not happening presently. This statement might help you become aware that, presently, you are unharmed.

"No matter what happens, I can handle it." This

phrase makes you aware of your internal resources and motivates you to overcome life's problems. This idea is from the tradition of Cognitive Behavioral Therapy

"I am responsible for my problems. Can I put an end to it? The first section of this phrase originated from the Four Noble Truths of Buddhism. A few times, I say to myself "I am responsible for my problems! Again!!" I use this phrase so often that I now have shortened it to, "responsible for own problems." This helps me save time.

The second part of the phrase, "Can I put an end to it?", has its origin from motivational studies advising that you are more likely to be encouraged by asking yourself a question, rather than saying, "I can put an end to this", or judgmental - "Avoid causing more problems for yourself" - this only creates additional problems. The simple question, "Can I put an end to this?" makes you aware that it is up to you to make that choice. Definitely, if there is actually an unfortunate event likely to happen, perhaps a death in the family, a divorce, or a natural disaster, the ideal thing to do will be to ask yourself, "What is the best thing to get ready in case this ever happens?". Making preparations for your action plan can be a relief for worry.

If you are responsible for your own problems by asking yourself "what if questions", admit these thoughts, comfort yourself with one of those statements as mentioned earlier, and then keep moving. If you discover that your thoughts are wandering to your favorite tragic thoughts, do not be discouraged. Making changes to your thinking habits might be difficult and lapses are expected. In reality, controlling tragic thoughts is a project that can last through a lifetime. Yet, positive self-affirmations can help you overcome the "what if's" very quickly, so that you can concentrate your thoughts on the things that are important to you.

What to Do When Considering The Worst-Case Scenario

Since I am a true child of my mother, thinking of the worst possible scenario comes naturally to me. How can we prevent this, since that kind of thinking is ingrained in our DNA?

So....

- **Be aware that your worst, is only your worst.** What you regard as your worst possible scenario is exclusively based on your personal experiences and knowledge. Strictly speaking, there is always someone that is facing a more terrible situation. So, your worst might not even be the worst possible scenario.

- **Know that you do not know the worst. Don't believe you know the worst.** A long time ago, my mother told me that she created the worst possible scenario that can happen. And like I told my mother, it is difficult to come up with ALL the possibilities. Stop trying to, it is just impossible.

- **Re-channel your energy.** It can be very draining

to come up with all the worst possible scenarios. If you expend so much energy on thinking, there is no energy left for actually taking action. So channel your "What if?" energy into concentrating on taking steps.

- **Come to terms with the worst.** The worst can take place and it can be terribly awful. You are not learning if you are not hurt. So if the worst case takes place, come to terms with it and learn from it.

Why You Should Consider the Worst-Case Scenario

Sometimes when we get to the root of our utmost fear, we become aware that it is not so scary. If you are forced to become innovative, your suffering can yield positive results, create a solution, and help overcome your challenges.

There are some reasons why this is effective for a lot of people:

- **It enables you to come back to the present moment.** Most times when we feel scared, it is because we allow our brain to run wild with all the possible scenarios. Thinking about the worst possibility and coming to terms with it helps to bring you back to the present moment.

- **It creates the space needed to assess your thoughts and weigh the possibilities.** When we assess those things that are very important to us, we can provide an explanation for the fear by asking ourselves, "What are the possibilities that this thing I am scared of will actually happen?" You can also assess your thoughts thoroughly with some basic questions.

- **Eventually, it enables you to process, certain that even if the worst comes to pass, you will still be fine.** For a lot of "ifs," we simply want to know that the next step we take will not drive us to the darkest parts of the Earth. When we assess the worst possibility, taking that next step will be easier.

Eventually, we are all making attempts to guarantee our safety and our physiological stress response is an excellent tool. Although, it is important to assess the stress to be sure that the worst possibility is actually the worst and the best thing to do when facing problems is to come up with solutions.

Learn to move according to the flow, surrender to the wind, turn to the side, and take charge.

Chapter 6: Schedule Thinking Time.

Thinking and overthinking are two different things. Thinking is the process of considering ideas, actions, and the likes. It is a process of examining and pondering on possible reactions, actions, or ideas. This act is very important and essential before decision making. It might not be so easy to control how, when, and what to think about but this is very achievable through constant practice. Practice will always make perfect.

As important as thinking is, we still have to be in control of what we think about, when we think and how frequent we do it. Leaving our minds to choose our thinking times for us might not be so healthy as we will be thinking at random. One way we can prevent this is by scheduling our thinking time to a more comfortable period and sticking to it.

The thinking process is more suitable during the day than at night. This is because our minds need rest, and the perfect time to rest the mind is at night, while we sleep. Therefore, instead of keeping the mind busy at night, use it during the day to think and sort out certain problems. This will help you to have a perfect night's rest. However, when it comes to fantasizing about something, the most suitable time to do this is at night and not during working hours when you need to concentrate.

Overthinking is a habit formed over time and to change it can take a while. It is a multifaceted process that requires a lot more than just saying words of determination. You have to be determined in your actions and scheduling thinking time is one of those actions you can take.

The "Schedule Thinking Time " Steps.

Scheduling thinking time can look very abstract for beginners but it gets better with consistency. There are steps involved in doing this. Below are the steps or guidelines you need to follow. No matter how foolish the following steps look, do not stop the exercise.

1. Select a reflection process that matches your preferences. There are many ways we can reflect on things, some of these ways are: having a diary, opening to someone you can trust, taking a walk, and lots more. If one way does not seem achievable, then try another but have time to meditate. When we have problems, we should not wave them off with incessant talks about sports, news, and fashion. Talking about these things are not bad but when they take our reflection time, it becomes a problem.

2. Schedule thinking time each day for one week. Form the habit of thinking at a time every day for at least a week. For a start, it can be a minimum of 15 minutes, usually in the morning hours or in the day. Your thinking time should not be at night just when you are about to sleep. This is because it will keep you awake and you won't get enough sleep required by the body.

3. Start small. As a beginner, you don't have to force yourself with one-hour reflection time if you cannot stick to it. Scheduling thinking time is a process. It is one thing to schedule thinking time, it is another thing to stick to it. Therefore, start small, it can be 10 minutes or less, as far as you can stick to the time.

4. Don't plan what you are going to think about. Let this appointment with yourself be totally unplanned. Do not set aside the exact thing you are going to think about and do not schedule your time to fall under the days or periods that you have lots of work to do. There should be no agenda for this meeting, let it be a time of surprise for you and your thoughts.

5. During that 15-30 minutes window, write down all the thoughts you have. Before your thinking time every day, determine that you will not worry or overthink about the thoughts you are about to have, until the next thinking session. This will help you keep your thoughts in check even after the thinking time.

Sometimes, we might not know what is bothering us but with this step, these things will be revealed. It is advisable that during our thinking hours, we should try to put down the thoughts we had. This will help to give us a clearer view of what is bothering us and what is not. Before your thinking time elapses, if your mind should lead you to the possible solutions to your problems, then it's fine, but if not, do not think about the problem outside your thinking window.

6. Between thinking times. Do not think about your thoughts during the last thinking time until the next. This means that you should not worry about your problems or the solutions to them outside your thinking time. This is not as easy as it sounds, you will require deliberate actions to stop yourself from worrying over certain issues at random. Determine strongly within you to worry about your problems only during your scheduled thinking time.

7. At the end of the week, take a few minutes to look at what you wrote down over the course of that week. At the end of every week, take out time to look at your thoughts over the week. Notice the recurring thoughts, the thoughts that stopped coming after a while, the ones that kept coming, the changes in your thoughts, and every single detail of your thought patterns. Meditate on these discoveries as this will help you to pick out the first ten on your list.

8. Doing this for one week, consider trying it for another. Remember practice makes perfect, a habit is not formed in a day, but consistency makes it happen. Practice the above steps more often and you will realize over time that you are in control of your thoughts, where, when, and how often you think.

The thinking process is very essential as mentioned earlier; it is one of the active problem-solving measures. It is one of the ways of dealing with life's uncertainties. This life is full of risks, we cannot predict what will happen in the next 30 minutes and this has caused a lot of people to resolve to worry about every little thing. However, instead of giving yourself to all the causes of worries in life, you can think about the ones you can solve and let go of the ones you cannot.

Train your mind to remain calm and peaceful around situations.

Chapter 7: Think Usefully.

The majority of us are fond of overthinking situations that we really can do nothing about. To be honest, it is totally pointless to keep thinking of these things. I will strongly recommend that you start thinking effectively.

For example, you have been looking forward to a promotion at work. You have to remember that getting that promotion is TOTALLY in the hands of your employer, no matter what extra qualifications you add to your resume. Useless thinking, in this case, is a waste of time and mental energy wondering if he will promote you or not.

On the contrary, your thinking should be centered on what you need to do in order to qualify for a promotion. You might need to up your skills, or get another certificate, or even show more dedication to your job. Whatever the case may be, think to produce results, not to lament!

I do agree that it is not easy to break some thinking habits, but freeing yourself from these patterns can unlock the ingenuity in you and I have here various ways to help free yourself from these thinking patterns.

Test theories. There are essential suppositions for every new case. You should test these theories for a wider variety of opportunities and prospects.

You presume that you cannot afford to purchase a house or even make a deposit, so you don't buy the house based on this presumption. Test that theory by evaluating your assets to see if their worth can get you that house in exchange. I mean, you may not have the money in cash or in your account but don't take a huge action based on a presumption. Ask yourself what you can do to get the money and maybe it won't look as impossible.

Paraphrase the issue. You might be surprised to find that you become innovative when you say it differently. You can only achieve this with an open mind and looking at the issue with different perspectives. Try to look at it from the outside, without sentiments, so you can attack the problem logically. Ask yourself all the hard but important questions and it will be easier to hatch new plans to fix the issues.

In the mid-'50s, enterprises that owned shipments lost their cargo on wagons. Even though they later tried to target more rapid building and development, and more efficacious ships, they still cannot fix the issues. Soon, a specialist changed the description of the issue, talking about it a whole other way. He suggested that evaluating the ways the industry can start decreasing the cost should be the new dilemma. This new direction of focus opened doors to new strategies. Every area not excluding the shipments and storage was deliberated upon. Eventually, the result of this new focus was what is called a container ship and roll on wagon/crate.

Flip your thoughts. When you get stuck and can't get around an issue, try inverting it or doing a flip flop on it. Take it from the other end. Consider how to create the issue and aggravate the situation, as opposed to deliberating on how you can fix it. This reversal strategy will create novel tips on how to go about the case. When you then turn the matter upright, you might get clarity.

Use various ways to communicate. We don't always have to use our verbal logical medium in the face of a problem which we are quite typical of. We are too smart to limit our reasoning capabilities. Use other methods to articulate the issues. At this point, don't worry too much about resolving the matter. Just articulate. Various people with various means of articulation can come up with many new thinking patterns to breed new ideas.

Connect the dots. It seems like most of the most effective ideas are never planned, they just happen. It may be something random you saw or heard that inspires you enough to birth that smart idea. There are many examples to support this - Apple, Newton, and so on.

You might wonder why we are affected by randomness in such a manner, it is because these unpredictable things trigger our brains into new thought patterns. Hence, you can use this to your advantage and link the disconnected segments.

Deliberately hunt for an impetus even in surprising places and try to link the disconnected pieces of the case and the impetus. Ways to build the network are:

Use unrelated tips. How about randomly picking a word from the dictionary and trying to create a network between your issue and the word.

Associate the probable ideas. Put a particular word on the page, write everything that comes to mind on that same page. Then try to create a network between them.

You can randomly take a photo, for instance, and see how you can link it to the case.

Pick up something, anything, and consider how it can contribute to your case positively by asking yourself vital questions to figure out what the item has as a feature that can help turn the situation around.

Change your outlook. If you want fresh ideas, you may need to change the way you see the situation because as time goes on, having a particular point of view will only result in the same associated ideas.

Ask for another's opinion. People are so different, we all have different ways we will approach a situation. Hence, ask other people for their opinions and their preferred line of action on the case. It can be a child, or a friend, patron, your partner, or even a random stranger with another lifestyle entirely and perhaps a completely different outlook to life.

Indulge yourself in a game. You can attempt to see things from a millionaire's point of view for instance, or ask yourself what Obama will do if you were him.

Any notable person you might choose has a distinguishing character, therefore, consider these attributes and use them to approach the issue from another angle. For example, if you take on the millionaire role, then you may have to display their attributes too when strategizing. Attributes like an extravagance and adventurous business. Someone like Tiger Woods, on the other hand, will be more likely to display perfectionism, tenacity, and close observation to every nitty-gritty of the case.

You won't just need to plan a facultative design, but you will also want to practice all the tips mentioned above. The facultative design you come up with can aid in building up an optimistic feel, which then improves your innovative thinking.

Every time you feel yourself drifting into overthinking mode, direct your thoughts towards effective thinking and do away with any thinking that is not productive.

Chapter 8: Set Time Limits for Making Decisions.

Everything about us is because of our decision making. The friendships, the health, or even our vocation and every other thing that makes us who we are today are our capacity or incapacity to make decisions, and the choices we have already made. That said, it is unfortunate that a lot of people still find it hard to make decisions. Even if everything else seems to be going well for us, when the chips are down and the time calls for it to make that judgment call, we curl up. It just seems so hard to decide on something and stick to it.

Every single day, we live by the innumerable decisions we have to make, minute or huge. That is what life is all about. Progress will be more attainable if we can break down these huge decisions into little decisions.

The statement that the best decision is no decision at all, is almost always inaccurate. Indecisive people are more likely to be controlled by their lives instead of the other way around. With no control over your life as a result of indecisiveness, you may not be as self-sufficient as you will like, thus, you need to learn to be decisive and take charge of your life.

The best way to instigate your overthinking habit is to have a decision to make with a need to get it right and more than enough time to make it. The whole process of contemplating the best step to take, considering all your options while taking your time, is just an invitation to overthinking things. Setting a time limit for yourself is really the most effective way to curb that habit. It is advisable to set a limit with the span based on the severity or magnitude of the decision. Ensure that you halt all additional evaluation once the limit is reached and just select an option, act on it and proceed.

The purpose of this advice is to leave no chance for overthinking and enforce action through your set time limit. It is quite easy: simply start timing yourself just as you start the analysis process to make a decision. Because of your consciousness of time, your analysis of the advantages and disadvantages will be more concise. In fact, this technique is so easy and doable.

If you take too much time to make decisions, then this advice is just what you need. You can set the time as short as 1 min, or as long as 5 mins, or any number in between.

How to Set Time Limits For Your Decisions

- **Set a bar on your number of options.** While trying to make a decision, cut down your options to at most 3 things, as opposed to leaving your options wide, vast, and unlimited.

- **Parkinson's Law (set a bar on your time).**

When you set a time limit, it makes you work less, and stress your brain less and there will simply not be enough time to accomplish working your brain out. Work will only move to use up the available time.

- **Keep your opinions to the minimum.** Three people to offer their opinions is enough to help you with your analysis. Don't cause confusion for yourself, people are different, the less contradictory opinions you get, the easier it will be to come to a conclusion.

Reminder: if you find that you persistently ask for the opinions of others, then it might indicate that you may not be so sure of what you want, or you may just not want it at all. Getting a second or third opinion once in a while can help you verify a decision you most probably have already made.

- **Napkin technique.** Because you can't do much on a napkin, it's best to draw out your plan on a napkin first and you will find that only the most important things will be drawn.

- **Be positive.** When you learn to see the positivity in every option and decision, then you will be able to accept the consequences either way, without regret. You make the decision and then learn from it.

- **Walk the plank technique.** Make yourself vow to do something you hate or would rather not do if you don't make a decision within your stipulated time. You either go all the way or not go at all.

Set A Limit To The Number Of Decisions You Make Per Day.

To curb overthinking, give your brain enough time and space for when you have crucial decisions to make, by cutting down on the less important decisions. It is easy to get it wrong by thinking that cutting down on decisions is similar to cutting down on expenses but you can't be further from the truth. The truth is that the time, no matter how seemingly short it is, to make those less crucial decisions can stress your brain out before you even bring up the more critical ones, reducing the mental capacity of your brain for that moment. Therefore, it is best that you delegate those little decisions while saving up that mental energy for the crucial decisions. So save your brain the stress!

This is especially referring to those little daily tasks you need to decide upon but are not particularly crucial.

It is a known fact that Steve Jobs repeated the same clothes every single day just so he will not have to ponder on what clothes to put on daily. Just so Tim Ferris can avoid wondering about what to eat every morning, he has the same kind of breakfast, albeit healthy, every single morning. President Obama too restricted his replies on email to either "agree", "disagree", or "discuss" in order to dis-involve his mental energy from these little decisions.

Hence, from now on, when considering the tasks to assign, ensure that the mental energy they cost is well evaluated.

Therefore, we can safely say that less overthinking translates to more personal growth and development.

Reducing the weight of your decision making will always pay you no matter how you choose to go about it. You may employ a virtual assistant to take care of all your managerial tasks, or hire a freelancer to take care of one or two things as the needs arise, nonetheless, delegation pays.

Put a deadline on your thoughts. Limit your number of daily decisions and set short time-limits for decisions.

Chapter 9: Consider the Bigger Picture.

Overthinking only magnifies trivial things so much it causes panic, and the world is already terrifying enough as it is. Also, overthinking makes a little issue an unnecessarily big deal.

Every day, we go through one trial or the other and over time, our bad experiences breed fear. Fear of bereavement, or loss of valuables, fear of dissatisfaction and discontentedness in life, fear of flopping in an interview and losing a job you have not even gotten yet, or fear of ruining that first date.

Don't let yourself be limited and held down by fear. Don't let fear keep you from reaching the heights you desire.

Not everything will go as planned but don't be discouraged because setbacks usually are indicators of greatness yet to unfold. Hence, when making your plans, you need to learn to relax and trust the process. The relationship between intention and fear is the tendency to be less afraid when we are more willing to believe in our intentions and push aside every negativity to focus on the chances of having good end results.

Overthinking is so easy. It's so easy to let yourself slip into that over-analytical mode every single day but you need to learn to pause and look at the general overview.

We need to realize that most of these things that seem like a big deal now will most likely not be significant in a few months, or a few years, or sometimes even in a few weeks.

The moment it dawns on you that what seems so huge of a deal is only but a minute speck in comparison to the broad view, then maybe you will stop magnifying it.

Outlined below are a few tips to clarify things and help you look beyond your fears to see the general overview:

- **Pause and ruminate.** Immediately when you start to feel yourself overthink, just pause for a moment to mull over things. Then asking yourself plain but important questions might help put things in perspective.
    - **Ask yourself what the issue is precisely.** Identify the specific problem you are having a hard time with is and this can help you make the right adjustments.
    - **Ask yourself about how the whole thing makes you feel.** If you find yourself unsettled over it, then you most probably won't get any clarity.
    - **Now ask yourself about the why.** Why did you respond the way you did? Was your reaction suitable? You will agree with me that we tend to lose it and have a fit in the face of a volatile situation. Pausing to consider these things can help get issues clarified.
- **Come to terms with the things you can do**

nothing about. It is pointless and enraging to overthink things that you can't change and it can cause you to have a mixed up view of life. It can be hard but with the tips below, you can learn to just let go of things you can't control.

- **Identify your part and task.** Can you do something about it? Or is it totally out of your control?

- **Be optimistic.** One of the few ways to handle a case you have no control over is to just find something good about it and stay optimistic.

- **Progress.** Retrace your steps when you find that you are going around in a circle, getting the same outcome. Assess your actions to consider other options.

- **Stop measuring yourself up against other people.** Comparing your occupation, appearance, skill, and wits to those of others is totally uncalled for. Life influences and molds people in different ways and no two people have the same lives. These comparisons only set unattainable heights for yourself to reach. Nobody else has lived your life but you and you can never live another's life. Never forget that you are one-of-a-kind.

- **Learn from past experiences.** No matter what you might be combating, reflect on past events in relation to the issue at hand and watch yourself worry less. So, deliberate on the lessons to be learned from these historical events and see how they can help solve the issue at hand.

- **Concentrate on the things you can change.** It's harder to make changes to a case you deem impossible. Therefore, start by trying to change the littlest things in your control in order not to feel totally useless. For instance, when job hunting is looking futile, try to pinpoint what you should do to begin or accelerate the process. Sooner than later, you will find more jobs to apply for or just simply fill an application form to begin the process.

- **Be hopeful about the future.** Another thing that overthinking does, is make the future look bleak to you. You might just feel like there is nothing to look forward to. You need to learn to separate the current happenings in the present from the unknown in the future. Your pessimism in the present doesn't have to take away the hope of the future, no matter what. Instead of saying things like "I will never be able to complete this work", say "how can I achieve this goal and complete my work." See yourself done with the project and look forward to the satisfaction.

- **Pinpoint your feelings.** Your tendency towards optimism may sadly be dependent on how other people see you. Be concerned on how you view yourself, and who you are to you instead of caring about everyone's perspective of you. For instance, be more quick to ask yourself what you like in yourself instead of what they may or may not like about you.

- **Never forget that things change.** Life is variable. Times and seasons change. Those who are happier and sometimes live longer are those who have learned to adjust to those changes. For a clearer understanding, one way you can learn to adjust is by seeking out old pictures and noting how much you have grown. Perhaps you can start all over again by taking photos of yourself now as a measure against the change you desire. Looking at the "basis" picture from time to time can inspire you and help you to work on the present.

- **Visualize your surroundings.** You should be comforted knowing that in this vast world, there are, most likely, at least 2 other people who have a similar issue to yours. You are not alone! Stop trying to solve every problem, the truth is that you are only one being, you can't win them all by yourself.

- **Devise practical objectives.** Setting up reachable goals can really help sustain clarity. When setting up your goals, stay away from unrealistic goals, those ones that are so daunting, they seem impossible. For instance, you can set a goal where you will lose a few pounds per month if your long term goal is to be 100 pounds slimmer. Instead of trying to lose it all in the first few months, break it into units.

Put things into a wider perspective. Ask yourself how long this will matter. Will this matter in 5 years? Or even in 5 weeks? Envision a happy ending.

Chapter 10: Live in the Moment.

Life is like a moving train; it does not wait for you to be certain about your future before joining the ride, neither does it wait for you to get over your past. Life is made up of the past, the present, and the future but we are given a precious gift of the present every day. The past is just there to remind us where we have been and the future, to remind us of where we are going but the present is the life we are living already. Getting choked up with our pasts can make us forget the life we are supposed to live, making time pass us unnoticed. Life is precious, we can only live it in the present, not the past and not the future either.

It is not unusual to face challenges, distractions, hurts, and other negative things such that we prefer to hide in the shadow of our past instead of facing reality. This is not going to help anyone anyways. Most people just exist without living, they go about their schedules like puppets without really having time to enjoy the present. They go about it with smiling faces but unhappy eyes just because they are stressed and obviously need a break, a break to go on that vacation, to sit doing nothing, to just be free.

Despite our tight schedules, we should always try to live in the moment, this is also known as mindfulness. Mindfulness is the state of being totally aware of the present. Being mindful is accepting your thoughts as they are without worrying too much about them. It is being aware that life must be lived, not just existing. A mindful person will always live not based on his/her thoughts and this is who you should be.

Why Is It Important To Be Present?

Living in the present helps you to appreciate life more. It prevents you from remaining in the past or overthinking about the future. Living in the present is a skill that must be acquired to help you live a more exciting life.

Below are some of the important things about living in the moment.

- **Less worrying and overthinking.** Living in the moment or being present keeps you fully aware of the now. It prevents you from worrying and overthinking about the future and remaining in the past.

- **You can appreciate the world a little more.** When you live in the moment, you tend to appreciate the world around you. You won't be working yourself up over the past and fear for the future.

- **You can find out what might be bothering you easily.** Sometimes, you might not know what is bothering you but living in the moment or being present will help you realize when you are not doing so fine, emotionally, physically, and otherwise.

- **You may start to feel more relaxed.** Being in

the present enables you to be in control of your life and this will help you to feel more relaxed. Once you feel you are in control, you won't be too worried about life.

Practical Steps To Living In The Present.

Some people live their lives in the past, while others live theirs in the future. However, the past has gone, the future is yet to come, the only true moment we have is the present. So always live in the present because that is where we can really live.

1. Remove unneeded possessions. Getting rid of some items that remind you of your past can help you move on and you will be able to live in the present. Get rid of anything that keeps reminding you of the past.

2. Smile. Just smile. It does not just brighten your day but that of others as well. Every new day is a gift and we should always welcome it with a smile. Life can be full of uncertainties but you can control what happens to you. So, keep a positive mindset towards life.

3. Fully appreciate the moment of today. Each day is a blessing so make memories, appreciate nature, notice every detail of the day, don't allow any time to pass unnoticed.

4. Forgive past hurts. Keeping malice doesn't hurt

anybody but you. Try and forgive all those who have wronged you in the past. Don't have any reason for the past to haunt you, let all hurt go by forgiving.

5. Love your job. You don't have to keep doing what you hate for 5 days out of 7 days a week. This is the highest level of time wastage and it should be stopped. You can either quit the old job completely and look for something else that you love or you can focus on a particular area in the old job that you love and be able to do with joy.

6. Work hard today, but don't stop dreaming about the future. Don't let dreaming about the future take over living now. Don't live in a dream and forget about your reality. Dreaming about the future, having goals and aspirations is not enough to give you a golden future. You must work hard now to achieve these goals.

7. Stop dwelling on past achievements. If you find yourself dwelling or talking about your past achievements too much, then it is as a result of little or no achievements in the present.

8. Acknowledge and observe your worries. Don't try to overlook your worries, don't even try to control them. However, acknowledge your worries, consider them from a stranger's point of view without having to respond to them.

9. Let your worries go. When you don't dwell on your worries, they will be waved away as quickly as they came. Learn to let go of your worries, don't fix your mind on them.

10. Stay focused on the present. Our emotions,

thoughts, and feelings change constantly. So, ensure that you are moving with the change, once you realize that you are thinking about a thing for too long, call yourself back to the present. Consciously always try to live in the present moment.

11. Think beyond old solutions to problems. Our world is constantly changing; rules are changing and so are solutions to problems. Don't get used to the old ways of doing things, be open to change and accept it. The approach you use to solve a problem today might not work for the same problem tomorrow. Don't allow any time or moment to pass you unnoticed. This will enable you to always live in the present.

Spend more of your time in the present moment. Slow down. Tell yourself: Now I am... Disrupt and reconnect

Chapter 11: Meditate

Overthinking will not clear your mind, neither does it help you come up with a practical solution. Instead, it results in spiteful, redundant, and obsessive thinking. It is likely for the logical thinking process to be obscured by an overthinking mind. You are aware that it is impossible to change the past and no one knows the future. Still, the mind is embedded in a web of thoughts. Do not forget that there is a thin line between understanding your past mistakes and being obsessed about them.

Observing a child can help you discover that in the mind of a child, only 'today' exists. There are no thoughts concerning the future, or the past, they just enjoy what is currently going on. We were once children. And we have the ability to live in the present and avoid the stress of overthinking. How? You may want to ask. Not only does meditation help you stop overthinking, but it also takes you back to the times when everything was simple.

Meditation is an excellent way to absolutely prevent overthinking. Take a seat on a serene place, concentrate on your breathing, and consider clearing out every thought from your mind. When a thought drops into your mind, regard it without any emotional involvement, be aware of the thought but do not allow it to impact you.

4 Ways in Which Meditation Helps

To Stop Overthinking

Re-orient your objectives. Your mind can be overburdened with redundant ideas and thoughts when you overthink. You can be stressed by regrets, suspicions, doubts, twisted reality, and allusions. All these will not help you to live happily or calmly. You become aware that your thoughts are skewed and constructive. If you are prepared to know more, you will be able to put it all together to carry out the bigger quests in life.

Fights against negative thoughts. Most times, we shift the blame for all the problems in our life. At least, dealing with problems is simpler when there is another person to blame. Meditation helps you fight against unhealthy habits, like blame-shifting and fault-finding. Try out mindful meditation. It is highly effective in preventing you from overthinking. In this space of awareness, you will be able to seek real truths and get rid of toxic thoughts. Thus, helping you to concentrate on positive deeds and thoughts.

Declutter your mind. Overthinking is a key signal that something is eating you up. Get to the root of your apprehension and fix it squarely. One of the beneficial effects of meditation is that it declutters your mind. You are able to strategize, arrange, and make effective analysis in your mind. As soon as you understand the problem, you can start thinking of how to deal with it. This helps to prevent wandering thoughts, which can be unnecessary and toxic.

Detaches you from attachment. Overthinking is an

expression of all that you are bound to - your thoughts, words, ideas, and actions. There is too much attachment between us and other people, or us and relationships, this blurs our thinking and judgment, making us over-analytical and overly critical.

However, this is what you need to know about meditation, there is no one way to do it, there is no wrong or right way. At the early stages, meditating feels weird. Certainly. Your head will provide you with a long list of how it is a waste of time. What is the point of sitting there without thinking of anything? You will twist and turn. You will become angry. Persevere through it all. It becomes easier.

How to Meditate In 9 Simple Steps

1. Dedicate 5-30 minutes every day. As a beginner, start with five minutes. For a lot of people, five minutes is ideal, and actually, five minutes of meditation can have positive effects. Regarding frequency, it is believed that meditation should be a daily goal, like brushing teeth.

2. Get rid of distractions. Select a period of the day when you have a minimal amount of distraction. Perhaps, during the early hours of the day.

3. Relax and get comfortable. Before meditating, a few people enjoy stretching because it helps relax and loosen up your muscles. Sitting still might be hard as a newbie; however, stretching and relaxing gives you a head start.

4. Select your position. It does not matter if you are sitting up or lying down, your position is a personal decision. For some people, lying down is comfortable, for others, sitting up is. The key thing here is to be comfortable, that is not slouching, and with the spine straightened. If you are sitting, relax and place your hands over your lap. Sitting cross-legged on the floor while being supported by a cushion, or on a chair and place your legs on the ground. It is not compulsory to contort your body into a lotus position if it will be uncomfortable.

5. Concentrate your thoughts. Get ready for the meandering of your mind. The secret to meditation is to focus your mind on what is happening presently and not on what has happened, or what will happen in one hour. Now, you have to be still, relaxed, and simply heal yourself. As soon as you have selected the ideal period and you are relaxed and comfortable, you will be prepared to concentrate your mind on your breathing. It is a personal decision whether you want to meditate with your eyes closed or open. Sometimes, relaxing music can help you meditate effectively. If you enjoy meditating while listening to music, that is acceptable. There is a variety of music to listen to.

6. Take slow, deep breaths. Gently close your eyes. Start by breathing slowly and deeply - inhale through your nose and exhale through your mouth. Avoid breathing forcefully. Allow it to come naturally. The initial air intakes might be shallow but as you let your lungs fill with air each time, your breaths will progressively become fuller and deeper. You can take all the time you require to breathe deeply and slowly. After a while, the deep breaths start to make you feel more relaxed and at peace.

7. When your mind wanders, focus it back on your breathing. It is to be expected that your mind will wander. Gently try to focus it back to the present, that is, your breathing. Your thoughts might drift away as much as every five seconds. This is perfectly fine. Once you start to practice meditation frequently, there will be a reduction in the wandering of your mind and your body and mind will actually relax. Sitting quietly and concentrating on your breath is difficult but make that subtle deliberate effort to focus your mind on the present. This is the concept of meditation - focusing your awareness on what is presently happening. Additionally, if you think you might fall asleep, switch up your position.

8. Ending your meditation. As soon as you are prepared to end your meditation, open your eyes and stand up gently. Great work. You have done it!

9. Constant practice makes you perfect. It is not a competition. You might only be able to meditate for three minutes presently. Eventually, there will be an increase in this time, thus, an increase in all the beneficial effects of meditation. There is a significant difference with time. You will start to experience a feeling of happiness, peace, and calmness. Continue with it, it might be discouraging initially but that is fine. I am a multitasking, busy career mom, so it has been very beneficial for me. More beneficial than I imagined.

You can totally get rid of the bad habit of overthinking by meditating for 10 minutes each

day.

Chapter 12: Create A To-Do List.

Although your mind may be your strongest weapon; however, if neglected, your mind can also stop you from attaining your goals. Your mind tends to over exaggerate the true nature of things, making them larger than they actually are.

For example, if you have to finish a couple of tasks in one day, your mind might make it appear like an impossible feat to complete it in one day.

It comes up with multiple reasons the completion of the task will be impossible. The secret to avoiding this type of overthinking is to create a to-do list.

For example, if you have to create a presentation, complete a report, pick up your sister from the airport, or you have a meeting with a client, your mind might make it seem unimaginable to complete all these in one day.

Making a to-do list helps you assign a definite duration for each activity, making it simpler to complete them.

Here are a few ways to section these activities into a practical list, then cancel each activity once it is complete.

The Proper Way to Create and Complete a To-Do List

- **Select a method.** There are several varieties of a to-do list, so this depends on what is effective for a particular person. Some studies suggest that writing information by hand helps to recall it effectively;

however, if the last time you used a pen was 1995, do not worry; making a personal to-do list is also possible with the broad range of available digital apps.

- **Make several notes.** Make a few lists of tasks to be completed. There should be a master copy that has every task you want to complete in the long run. For instance, begin a language class, clear out the closet and so on. You can also create a weekly project list that has all the tasks that must be completed within one week. Then a third HIT list should be created, that is, High Impact Tasks list; this has a list of all the things that have to be done today - for instance, complete that work presentation, Call Uncle Tom for his anniversary, pick up the laundry. Each day, tasks from the overall list and the weekly task list will be moved to the HIT list, as appropriate.

- **Keep it simple.** Nothing is more terrifying than a long to-do list. In reality, it is impractical to complete such a huge number of tasks within 24 hours. One tip for simplifying the HIT list is to create a list of the tasks to be completed today and dividing it into two. The number of tasks on the list should be about 10, other tasks can be moved to the master draft or the weekly task list.

- **Begin with the simple tasks.** Before your MIT's, include a few basic tasks to the list: "Shower, Wash breakfast dishes, and fold clothes" are great examples. Completing and canceling out goofy tasks can help you start your day with a feeling of positivity.

- **Complete your MITs.** MIT stands for "most important tasks." The top of your list should begin with a minimum of two items that have to be completed urgently today, this is to ensure that you complete your project report that has to be submitted tomorrow, rather than vacuuming. Although the other tasks on the list might not be done, the very significant tasks will be completed.

- **Divide into smaller tasks.** Tasks like "work on thesis project" seems too imprecise and pressurizing, this implies that we might be too overwhelmed to actually start them. A great way to decrease fear and make the goal appear more realistic is to divide tasks into smaller projects. Rather than saying "work on thesis", be more specific, say something like "complete first half of chapter two" on Sunday and "write the second half of chapter two" on Monday.

- **Be specific.** The common qualities of all your to-do lists should be: they should be a task that can be exclusively completed by the creator of the to-do list, they are physical tasks, they can be completed in one sitting. For general tasks that need a great deal of time or assistance from other people, make a list of the specific steps that can help you achieve your goal. Rather than "rescue the animals," try out "create a cover letter for internship at World Wildlife Fund."

- **Include it all.** For all the things that have to be done on the list, be as expressive as possible, write everything concerning it so that there are no excuses if the job is not completed. For instance, if the task has to do with calling a friend, write that person's number on the list so that there will be no need for you to start looking for it later.

- **Time it.** Since you have created the list and cross-checked it two times, now set a time limit beside each task. Converting the to-do list into an appointment list might be helpful. For instance, clear out inbox 7-8 p.m. at Dominos on 5th Avenue, dry cleaning 8-9 p.m. at Clean Aces. Once the set time has passed, it has passed; spending seven hours picking up the dry cleaning is unnecessary.

- **Avoid stressing yourself.** Most master lists have one or two things that we have had the intention of completing for days, weeks, or probably years but we haven't gotten around to doing them. Try to come up with the reasons for this so that you can understand the steps required for the actual completion of the tasks. Avoiding the call to Aunt Jessie because of long hours that might be spent on the phone? Substitute "Call Aunt Jessie" with "find a way of ending the call to Aunt Jessie" This will lessen the varying extent of the task, making it easier to accomplish.

- **Share it with people.** A few times, the best way to remain obligated to do something is to have someone monitor us. You can make your to-do list public, by placing it on the refrigerator or creating a digital calendar that can be viewed by your colleague.

- **Fix a time to schedule.** Sitting down to create an actual to-do list might be one of the most difficult aspects of making the list. Select a time daily, maybe morning before everyone is up, or lunchtime, or even before going to sleep, when it will be easy for you to organize all that needs to be done and figure out what is still undone.

- **Go in with the old.** Reminding yourself about the past day's productivity is an excellent way to improve productivity. This carries a documented list of all the things you have achieved the previous day, including the silly tasks.

- **Make a new list.** Create a fresh list daily, so that constant old tasks do not overpopulate the list. Additionally, it is a beneficial way to ensure that we actually accomplish a task every 24 hours and do not waste time beautifying the list with colorful markers.

- **Be flexible.** Useful hack: Make sure to set apart 15 minutes of "compensation time" between tasks on the calendar or to-do list in case of an unplanned emergency; for instance, if your computer goes off or if there is an electrical short circuit. And if no unfortunate event happens, the most significant thing is to remember to hold off and breathe. If you have already completed at least one MIT - you will accomplish the rest.

Give a comprehensive detail of your projects and divide them into sections. Set a pseudo-deadline and see if they can be completed within half of the set time. Then eventually, fix a time for everything.

Chapter 13: Embrace Positivity.

The sad thing about life is that it is full of negative events. These events are often circulated around the world through the news, the social platforms, and the likes. As pathetic as this is, no one can control or prevent these things from happening. So, allowing these negative events to weigh us down is of no use because we cannot solve the problems. However, most people's mindset has been affected negatively by the unfortunate happenings around them. They end up over thinking about everything no matter how insignificant it may look.

You are not in control of what happens around you but you are in control of how you react to it or feel about it. Most people allow their mindset to be drawn to the negative side because of what they see or hear every day. When situations arise, we have two choices; to look at the negatives around the situations or to see the positives around it. Sadly, most people give in to the former. We are in control of our feelings, so you can either feed it with positive thoughts or negative ones.

Make a conscious choice to be optimistic about life. Embrace positivity. Get rid of anything that will make you unhappy and threatens your peace of mind. Overthinking brings doubt and, as a result, it leads to negative mindsets. Therefore, stop overthinking and be confident that you can overcome any storm that comes your way.

Consciously try to protect your peace of mind. You cannot

do this if you don't love yourself enough, if you think you don't deserve happiness. One thing is for sure, we all deserve love, we all have the right to be happy and, for all that it's worth, your happiness is your responsibility. Create happiness where it is absent, always give yourself a reason to be happy because you deserve it.

Nurse your mindset continually with positive thoughts. Despite the challenges you might face - the diverse feelings from pain to fear, anger, discouragement, and others - never stop thinking positive.

Below are some tips to help you embrace positivity;

- **Start on a good note.** Wake up every day feeling grateful. Be thankful for everything, think about the good things that happened to you the previous day, you can even jot them down. By doing this, you give yourself a good reason to be confident, to hope, and to be happy. This positive energy at the beginning of a new day is enough to keep you going for the whole day. Apart from the daily reflections, you can also try it on a weekly or monthly basis, this will help you maintain a positive mindset.

- **Notice the people you spend more time with.** Negativity is infectious, so watch the people you spend most of your time with. If they are always seeing the worst in everything, then you should reconsider hanging out with them. This is not because you hate them or you are judging them, you are just protecting your mind.

- **Speak positive words.** Just as our actions are

important, our words are too. In fact, the words we speak, over time, turn into our actions and become our reality. Watch the things you say; negative words will birth negative energy and eventually result in negative things. Our subconscious mind listens to us, it pays attention to what we say and do. After a while, it begins to respond to the words it heard, negative or positive. Therefore, always make positive statements.

- **Jog your memory.** We earlier mentioned living in the present and letting go of the past but there are some memories of the past we should not forget like memories of a happy childhood, a happy memory of the beach, and other happy moments. These memories give us the strength to live in the present. Therefore, create happy memories whenever you are given the opportunity.

- **Start to cultivate hope in small ways.** Create hope even in the smallest ways. It can be by seeing a smile on a stranger's face, by planning to achieve a goal, or by reflecting on the good things that have happened to you.

- **Shift your focus.** Stop trying to control everything. Loosen up a bit, shift your focus away from things that are not working and focus on the things that are.

- **Deactivate negative thoughts.** When you notice that you are beginning to have negative thoughts, do not nurture it but change it. When a negative event occurs, it can be an issue with parents or siblings or even a weight problem; do not think too much about it. Consciously prevent your thoughts from wandering to negative events; focus more on the positive ones.

- **Get back to basics.** It is not too late to change your mindset; it came as a result of thought. So, begin to have positive thoughts.

- **Be curious.** Don't assume you know everything. Think about the possible outcomes of events.

- **Think back to a time when you achieved something and what you did.** Never forget your achievements, the technique you used, and how you applied it. You may need to use the same procedure to achieve something greater.

- **Keep up the body talk.** Don't focus so much on the mind that you forget the body. When our bodies are healthy, our minds will also be healthy too. The state of our bodies will affect our minds, the physical body controls the activities of the mind to an extent. We all need a level of motivation each day and without the proper exercise of the body, we might not be able to get the positive energy we need. When we are physically healthy, we will be able to have a positive mindset towards life.

- **Start an evidence journal with proof that life is working out for you.** Record all the good things life has offered you, rather than the things it hasn't offered or the negative things it offered.

- **Think of someone whose life seems to be going well.** Do you have someone you wish to be like? Or do you admire a person's life? Then make them your role model, make inquiries about what they do and how they do it in order to be successful.

- **To err is human.** In a bid to embrace positivity, don't be too hard on yourself. Maintaining a positive mindset can be difficult. We are humans and we are likely to make mistakes, to have doubts and negative feelings but when they come, control them. Don't let them consume you, remember that feelings and thoughts do not last long, they will pass only if you don't nurture them.

Change your mindset and spend more time with positive people who do not overthink things.

Chapter 14: Using Affirmations to Harness Positive Thinking.

Most individuals who think negatively are those who often overthink. If you let yourself continue, soon, everything about you becomes negative and pessimistic; your self-esteem, your perspective, and your emotions.

The funny thing about negativity is how they seem to almost always come to pass. These negative thoughts depress your spirit, your relations with the people around you, and your personality. Somehow, you have convinced yourself that you will never be adequate and it is beginning to rule your life.

Be intentional instead, about being everything that is not negative; be optimistic and hopeful. Think and speak good words to yourself and you will find that it is very potent and beneficial.

Ultimately, make efforts to curb your overthinking habits by deliberately thinking more positively about life.

What Are Affirmations And Do They Work?

An affirmation is an assertion, an optimistic remark which really helps to inhibit negativity and self-damage. The more you declare these words, the more you actually believe them, and subsequently, the more positivity you can actually exude.

Constantly reiterating these words can help our mental state so much that it reforms our thought chains to make us start to think and behave positively.

For instance, there is proof that assertions aid in your work performance positively. When you are feeling a little nervous in anticipation of a big deal meeting, you can take a little time to focus on all your great attributes and this will help settle your nerves, improve your self-esteem, prevent you from being a nervous wreck, and increase the chances of your being productive.

Self-assertion can also ameliorate the terrible effects of anxiety and stress.

Even better, assertions have been a mental therapy for people suffering from depression, low self-confidence, and a plethora of other mental disorders. Assertions have also been proven to excite certain aspects of our brain that trigger the high possibility of being more positivity-conscious and directed concerning our health. When you have high regard for yourself, you become more concerned about enhancing your general health. Hence, if you think you eat too much, for instance, and need to start working out, then assertions can be used to help you remember your worth and, thereby, encourage you to make some lifestyle changes.

How to Use Positive Affirmations

Affirmations have no restrictions, you can use them whenever you will like to make positive alterations to your life. You can use them when you want to:

- Improve your self-esteem before crucial meetings and renditions.

- Command your emotions, putting a rein on any pessimistic feelings like anger, disappointment, and easy irritability.

- Revamp your self-assurance.

- Successfully end projects you began.

- Upgrade your efficiency

- Beat bad habits.

Affirmations work better with set goals and more optimistic thoughts.

Visualization complements affirmations quite perfectly. So, don't just visualize that great change, speak it to yourself, jot it down until you believe it. Positively assert yourself.

Affirmations are also very valuable when you are determining new goals and targets. The moment you specify exactly what you want to attain, self-assertion and affirmative remarks can aid in constantly driving you to success.

Saying those positive statements to yourself over and over again is really the key to potency. Paste it up on your wall, or set it as an alarm, but ensure you reiterate those words to yourself as often as possible every single day. Even more important is the need for you to reiterate those words when you find yourself overthinking again, or doing those habits you have been trying to break.

How to Write an Affirmation Statement

Your affirmation statement should be directed at a particular aspect or habit you are trying to break. You can customize your affirmation statement to your requirements using the tips below.

- Consider that habit you are trying to break away from. The behavior you want to improve on. It can be your bad temper or your easy irritability or your deficient communication skills or you're close to zero productivity at work.

- Next, jot down those aspects of your life that you will

like to make alterations to and be sure they align with your key values and every other thing that is vital to you. If you don't align these changes to your values, you may not be truly inspired to reach for those goals.

- Don't try to make impossible and unreliable affirmations, be realistic and practical about it. For example, you are not satisfied with the salary you get every month, you can start reiterating affirmations to yourself to raise your confidence enough to request for a raise.

- Nonetheless, it's best not to convince yourself that you will definitely get a raise double your previous salary because it is generally out of the question for employers to double your salary just like that. Be pragmatic and reasonable! It's not like affirmations are enchantments. What you need is belief, if not, those words might have little or no potency in your life.

- Switch up the negativity and embrace positivity. If you are fond of self-discouragement and general self-damage, learn to observe the particular thoughts or ideas that plague your mind. Then create an affirmation that completely contradicts that line of thought.

- Let's imagine that you frequently tell yourself that you are neither skilled nor talented enough to make any headway in your career, you can change this completely by writing an affirmation such as, "I am good enough, and I am a gifted expert at what I do."

- Be particular about writing in the present tense in a show of belief that what you are saying is taking place already. It's the only way for you to truly believe and see it truly happen. For example, a good example of an effective affirmation is, "I am ready for this presentation, I am well-versed in this topic because I have prepared well for it and it is going to be a wonderful presentation." Say this to yourself when you start to feel the nerves and anxiety over public speaking.

- Say it as if you mean it. Bringing emotions into your affirmation can really help you make the words more productive. If you truly want it, act like you do by saying it with volition. Say it like it makes sense to you and means something to you. For instance, if you are having issues with calming your nerves concerning a new project you were given, then try telling yourself something like, "I am looking forward to this new challenge. I can't wait to take it on".

Examples of Affirmations

By all means, your affirmation is exclusive to you, so let it specify exactly what you aim to attain and all the alterations you are looking to make. However, below are some examples that can help you start:

- My innovations for this new challenge are innumerable.
- My boss and all my colleagues will appreciate my work when I'm done.
- I have the capacity to get this done!
- My opinion is invaluable to my team.
- I am triumphant and victorious.
- Candor is my watchword.
- I am time-conscious about every task.
- I appreciate this job and do not take it for granted.
- I love accomplishing good work with my team.
- I am exceptional at everything I attempt
- I am magnanimous.
- I am fulfilled.
- I will set the pace in this company.

Affirmations are assertions of positivity that aid in defeating self-ruin and negativity in general.

Chapter 15: Become Action-Oriented.

You cannot just determine to stop overthinking but you have to deliberately take action to see that you are free from the habit. Don't think too much about making the right choice, we often learn from our mistakes. In fact, the best lessons are the ones learned from a mistake.

Always be ready to take action no matter how uncertain they may look. Overthinking brings doubts and these doubts restrict us from taking action where we should. One can never be too safe in life. Our lives will be a lot better if we can do most of the things we've had in mind to do.

However, when I talk about taking action, I mean directed action. Before you take any action, you must first consider it with the situation at hand, the action must be taken wisely and not based on emotions.

Tips to Taking Action in Overcoming Overthinking

1. **Acknowledge the outcome of the indecision.** The most effective way to get rid of overthinking is to identify the consequences of indecision. In every situation, compare the consequence of making a decision with the consequence of not making one. If the outcome of the latter is more favorable, then you must just move on.

2. **Flip a coin.** When it seems like you can't get your mind off an issue, it can be your instinct trying to warn you that the situation is either not under your control or that it is not necessary to overthink about the issue. All you need to do in cases like this is to open the next chapter and move on.

3. **Write 750 words.** Writing is one way you can employ to clear your mind. It helps you to clearly see what the problems are and devise ways to solve them.

4. **Decide twice.** Always test the strength of your decisions by trying to decide on that problem twice before taking action. After making a decision about an issue, write it down and after 24 hours, reflect on that same issue but this time around, in a different place. Then answer the same questions you asked yourself and make a new decision. Now, notice if it corresponds to the first decision.

5. **Trust your first instinct.** As earlier said, overthinking brings doubt. It restricts us from making decisions fast, it makes us lose faith or confidence in ourselves. Therefore, always learn to trust your first instinct.

6. **Limit the decisions you make.** You don't have to decide on everything. Learn to go with standards. This will limit the number of decisions you will have to make in a day and further increase your capacity to make better decisions for more serious issues.

7. **You can always change your mind.** Whatever gave us the impression that decisions must be very rigid, dominant, and severe? Decisions can be changed, one can have a change of heart at any time, this is what you need to know. You can decide now to buy a new property and decide later not to get it, it's all your choice and you owe no one an explanation. Your friends are only there to influence your decision and not make it for you. They can only try to talk you out of something but at the end of the day, it is your call. Good friends will always accept your decisions and support you all the way. However, when making decisions, choose exciting activities, things that make you happy. Remember your happiness is your responsibility.

There is something known as analysis paralysis. This is a condition caused by overthinking. It is a situation in which no decision is made about an issue because it has been overanalyzed.

Don't think too much about issues, it will only prolong them, rather, be a man of action.

Chapter 16: Overcoming Your Fear.

Letting feelings overcome us and shock us into overthinking is human nature. Who will walk right into a probably hurtful situation? Just that by consistently evading the "ghost" within, you will be a captive of the monster.

A very strong feeling is fear. It has a powerful impact on the mind and your physical appearance. It can establish powerful reactions when we are in alarming situations, for example, when in a fire or being assaulted.

Usually, this includes an attempt to combat any likely stressor that can lead to distress and involvement in limitless interruptions. But, you are combating possible situations that will bring you development and happiness. Additionally, you get to fight fear forever. Fear will attack no matter how hard you try to prevent it. And it will probably attack at a period when you require emotional composure the most.

Also, it can attack when you come up against nonlife-threatening situations such as dates, tests, new employment, a party, or facing a crowd. Fear is the usual response to a warning that can be sensed or evident.

These are a few recommendations to combat overthinking if you are encountering it:

- **Allow yourself to sit with your fear for 2-3 minutes at a time.** Inhale and exhale with the fear and state that, "It's fine, it looks very bad but feelings are similar to the sea - the tides ebb and flow." Ensure you have an uplifting activity planned for your post-sitting session: contact that confidant that wants to know how it went; dive into an activity that you find pleasing and intriguing.

- **Write down the things you are grateful for.** View what you've drafted out when you find yourself in a bad mood. Make the list longer.

- **Remind yourself that your anxiety is a storehouse of wisdom.** Draft a note, "Dear anxiety, I'm not afraid of you anymore, what can I learn from you?"

- **Use humor to deflate your worst fears.** For example, what are the worst funniest scenes that can occur if you honored an invite to speak to an audience of 500? I wet my trousers on stage. I can get detained for delivering the most horrible speech in the history of mankind, last boyfriend(girlfriend) will be part of the congregation and ridicule me.

- **Appreciate your courage.** Whenever you do anything that makes you afraid, despite the fear, you've made yourself a lot more powerful and the next attack of fear will probably not make you quit.

- **Reward yourself.** For example, When you call that person you really do not want to talk to, bolster your achievement by giving yourself something pleasing like a spa treatment, eat out, getting yourself a book, taking a walk, giving yourself something that gives you joy.

- **Change your view of fear.** If you are scared as a result of past failure, or you are just scared of doing something else, or you think the fact that you failed before means you will fail in other things, don't forget that the fact that you failed before does not guarantee that you will fail every time. Bear in mind that every moment is a new start, an opportunity to start afresh.

Don't get carried away by uncertain fears.

Chapter 17: Trust Yourself.

Being uncertain about yourself typically results in anxiety and overthinking things concerning tomorrow. You find that you lack the self-assurance to really manage specific plights and be decisive. Overthinking ensues because you feel deficient and you have misgivings about your own choices. Really, the issue with overthinking is how many commands your thoughts have over you. By and by, you start being skeptical about your ability to make wise decisions and ultimately lose trust in your decision-making skills.

Several people dwell in indecisiveness because they are hesitant to take charge of their lives, own up and bear the consequences of their actions. You jump at every opportunity to blame anyone else for the final decision they made on your behalf if events take a wrong turn. Nonetheless, the truth is that whatever decision was made about your life still comes back to you, especially if you acted on it. Because, as an adult, there are just some things concerning your life that you can't waive aside as someone's manipulative tactic over you. I tell you, it won't stand in court. You are responsible for your own life! Consequently, it is wise to learn to take account of every decision, step, and action you take.

In reality, no one can make you do anything. No matter how overbearing and controlling they are, you get to choose if you want to tow that line or not. Your actions or inactions remain your responsibility notwithstanding whose idea it was.

Instead of distributing your issues to be decided upon by other people, you can take control of your life by making your own decisions by yourself. Soon, you start to get a feeling of satisfaction and confidence in your judgments and their potential results. You need to get the hang of putting some credence in your capacity to manage specific scenarios. No one can believe in you as you will.

If you do not want to be held hostage by your overthinking, then you must get up and get things done in your life. You'll only be cheating yourself and miss out on potential self-growth and development.

Lucky for you, all you require to successfully manage every issue you encounter in your lifetime is confidence in your abilities.

Trust that you have the capacity to face anything life throws at you with the appropriate approach. The moment you begin to believe in your abilities, you start to overthink less and find yourself to be more decisive.

I will give you the scoop on what to do to learn to believe in your abilities:

- **Try not to overthink the end result of your judgment.** The world, in general, is variable and humans are hard to predict; hence, it would be preposterous to think that you can easily estimate the impending aftermath. As a result, we can say that decision making is almost always a shot in the dark. Although, trusting in yourself and your ability to make good calls is still very beneficial, know that you cannot control the end result of your decisions. Simply put, overthinking is pointless.

- **Try not to do things on a whim.** People tend to instantly be impulsive because they find thinking of the probable end result as an arduous task. Hence, they find it difficult to go through the deliberation process. Making an impulsive decision is not a terrible idea, in fact, over indecisiveness, it is an amazing idea. Nevertheless, with past experience of bad judgments, taking a little time to think about your decision is wise.

- **Face your fears.** People with no confidence in themselves are usually the ones that seek seemingly hassle-free routes. As a result of this lack of faith, they get scared of flopping and consequently, make bad calls. In the face of decision making, try to pick the choice you are most afraid of because that is your most likely path to growth.

- **Create a balance between paying heed to your sense of reasoning and trusting your gut.** Your best chance of having most of your decisions spot on is learning how to achieve an equilibrium between reason and gut feelings. Paying attention to only sense and rationale might just persuade you to go for the more prudent option as opposed to following your gut. You may even tell yourself that you need to wait for more information in that area before making any decision, and this can result in making no decision at all! Contrarily, following your gut can lead to you making careless calls. Therefore, paying attention to your whole self is crucial to making the right call especially concerning huge decisions. As they say, "don't forget to carry your brain along whilst listening to your heart."

- **Focus more on your past good decisions and the scenarios surrounding them.** Ask yourself how making that decision made you feel during and after making it and what you did to arrive at that verdict. Consider what made it a good call compared to whatever the other option was. Dwelling on your past good decisions will help you build confidence in your decision-making abilities knowing now that you do have these capabilities. Subsequently, you can easily unearth the most suitable game plan for your decision making. Personally, I have discovered that a sign that I'm making a good call is when I don't get hesitant while making a decision. When I trust in my decision is when I feel most organized and collected.

- **Make the choice that will afford you the most number of alternatives.** Everyone will like choices with lots of options to choose from. Albeit, there are choices that restrict you to a non-diverse set of options that will only be a strain on you later. You really don't have to go through the stress, so ensure you go for the option that is eventually going to be the most profitable choice, however hard it is to pick. Let your anticipation of the aftermath of your abilities trump that fear of failure.

- **Stop for a moment when faced with a tough call to make and ask yourself, "what if a miracle happened out of the blue and my whole life changes positively?"** This can ease the burden of what-ifs and help you see a possibility of good outcomes, hence, pointing you towards the better choice.

Rationality persuades us to take our time and get more information before we can deem ourselves ready to make a decision. This usually is as a result of our tendency to overthink things and fear making the wrong choices. It can leave us in a jam and with an unwillingness to take any action at all. You must know that indecisiveness in itself is already a made decision so it's essential to just go for it with a little of the rationale and a little guts to balance it. The moment you become more attentive to that inner voice which pops up from time to time to tell you what you truly desire, sense and rationality can then act in such a manner that will profit you in the long run.

Don't be scared of making blunders and errors because the truth is that many times, fear produces the best outcomes especially when you pick the option you are most scared of. There is a high probability of making the right choice you seek when it is really tough. Even though life is unpredictable, you must at least have dignity enough to be your own decision maker.

Tap into your nature neurons, trust your instincts, follow your guts.

Chapter 18: Stop Waiting for the Perfect Moment.

You are doomed to keep going round and round in a brooding loop of negativity if you let yourself overthink. It is depressing and pointless to keep lingering on the same thoughts. It doesn't even get better as overthinking can negatively influence you emotionally and mentally. Regrettably, several people are stuck with such idealism that they have completely lost touch with reality.

Overthinking gives you a semblance of a need for perfection but in reality, it just makes you dilly-dally on important matters.

For example, instead of just starting your business, overthinking will put you on pause whilst inventing unreal events in your head with questions like what if I do not have enough funds to start? What if time runs out before I can properly begin? What if no one wants to patronize me? Before you know it, you start questioning your preparedness.

At the end of the day, you may find that you never started the business.

However, how sure are we that the future will be brighter? Where's the proof? Can we really depend on our hope in the future?

Right now, this very moment, this present experience is what is certain, nothing else! The only certainty is the present. Let's face it, the probability of getting contentment from an unpredictable future moment is quite low especially if until now, you have still not had a fulfilling moment that really sated your unappeasable desires even after your great anticipation of it. So much for the proof of a brighter future.

We get too occupied with the past and the unknown yet awaited future. When our hope in the future for wealth and affluence fails us, we then turn to the past with sentiments on how things were before.

In our minds, is a euphoric place, somewhere with value, a brighter future, anywhere but where we are at that moment and somehow, we have belief in this place which we have told ourselves will bring us fulfillment and direction.

However, this utopia is only a figment of our imagination.

In reality, let downs and setbacks are what really ensues. Over time, as life proves itself to us as unable to hand out our blissful illusion of a utopia which quite honestly is being pushed by all kinds of media, we grow restless.

Every day, we grow more and more dissatisfied with life as we earn and acquire more, yet our real desires are not met. Soon, we start to feel more melancholic and dispirited, fidgety and apprehensive like there is a strain on us and subsequently, we start to act irrationally because we feel like the universe let us down. This doesn't help our friendships and relations with the people around us. Most times, a depressed man loses connection with everything that is real.

It is mental torture to keep holding your life to ransom in anticipation of a surreal moment when you want to be anywhere but where you are at the moment or be anyone but who you are presently. We seem to be stuck in fantasies we have created, all of which are dependent on that singular hope that there is something we can and should be doing in order to feel contentment in life.

How about we take a pause from everything and consider that we can find total and complete happiness in the present.

I can guarantee one thing; if you are willing to stop with the rapaciousness, then you will begin to realize that the here and now is just where you need to be to finally feel contentment.

The truth is that, notwithstanding the trials you face in life every day, every moment is precious and is how it should be. You need to start regarding life as it is.

Life is integral ephemerality and each second, each instant is but a piece of it. Time truly waits for no man and nature doesn't care about it. All we have are chains of splendid seconds and experiences which make up our entity. You must realize that you can only ever live once so these instants shared cannot be anything other than mere moments, so live in them, be aware of them.

For those who are still not inspired enough to quit the unnecessary brooding over what or what not the future really holds, need I remind you that there will come a day when you simply won't have the ability to worry. Whether you accept it or not, the hard truth is that death will most probably snatch you away before that illusion you have so perfectly created will materialize.

You can never retrieve those seconds you regretted or shunned. That time is gone forever! Appreciate every instant, seize the day, show yourself some love, show love to the people around you, and love the earth, it is your planet after all.

Make it a point to find contentment and happiness in each moment especially the here and now, don't just wave them aside. How you react to this present moment will greatly influence the next moment and subsequent moments after that. This has an effect on how many chances you get in life and how much wealth you ultimately amass.

Hence, live in the moment, whether you are enjoying or not enjoying every second, live in every moment instead of wishing for something spectacular to happen to you.

If you keep waiting for when you will be happy dependent on something specific happening, you may never be able to fill the hole of unfulfillment you have dug in your own heart. If nothing new has been able to satisfy you for long, then you know that I speak the truth. After a while, that new product doesn't do it for you anymore neither does that achievement or new date. You still feel empty and dissatisfied. You soon find yourself in a loop as you set yet another new goal and end up feeling the exact same way.

You need to begin to tell yourself that satisfaction and joy are neither waiting for you in some far away future nor has it overlooked you. It is right within your grasp in the here and now, in every passing moment. It's time to live in the moment and appreciate the beauty in every second, it's time to start living fully. This is it! It's already occurring, take what is yours!

No moment is more perfect than this one here, right now. There is no absolute moment. This one is going just how it should. Live it now.

Chapter 19: Stop Setting your Day up for Stress and Overthinking.

Completely escaping overpowering and overly stressful days is not possible but you can reduce the amount of these days per month or annually, by starting your day well and not preparing yourself for irrelevant stress, agony, and overthinking.

Three points that will aid with this are:

Get a good start. The way you begin your day, most times, creates the pace with which your day will run. A hard day will be a result of a stressful morning. Taking in bad news on your way to work will cause you to have negative thoughts all day.

Meanwhile, if you read a nurturing article during breakfast, doing a little exercise then starting your day with your most crucial task creates a great mood for your day and ensures you are optimistic all day.

Single-task and take regular breaks. This aids in maintaining an acute focus all day and to do the most crucial tasks. And at the same time creating room for relaxation and rejuvenation, so you do not run empty.

This kind of rested attitude with an acute focus will cause

you to think with clarity and precision, it will prevent tired and overthinking thought space.

Minimize your daily input. Excess news, continually checking your inbox and social media accounts, or the progress of your blog or website causes excess input and congests your head as the day gets by.

Hence, it is tougher to contemplate easily and with clarity, it will not be difficult to fall back into the well-known overthinking behavior.

Manage your peaks. Immediately you learn to locate important chores, you can plan how to get the maximum achievement. This is the part where we gather our innate strength.

We are well aware that once the job is moving steadily, distractions dissipate, our concentration is at its peak, and our job leaves us in awe; this is perfect. We certainly cannot neglect the vital (sometimes repetitive) chores that serve as maintenance for our companies, but we can notice when we are functioning in used time as against unused time.

If we are engrossed and battling crucial tasks at our maximum hours, we will want to work for more time and feel less tired as time goes on. Reducing our unused time can also maximize our strength and motivation and aid our concentration on crucial good thinking instead of unnecessary bad thinking. Immediately you have identified your peak periods, you are set to take advantage of these valued hours.

Get a good start. Single task and take regular

breaks. Minimize your daily input.

Chapter 20: Accepting Everything that Happens.

This is gotten from one of the lessons of stoic philosophy. The focus of this is that we are to accept whatever occurs, which can both be bad or good, and believe that it happens for the greater good even if it does not look like it at this moment.

Most times, overthinking occurs as a result of thinking on things that occurred in the past. We begin to imagine how circumstances will have been if things had not occurred the way they did. Depression often occurs as we continue to replay and overanalyze the situations in our minds.

Man's problems are a result of his thoughts he creates himself. The meaning of a thing is gotten from the meaning you give it. Your brain gives meaning to the events of life in order to make sense of what is going on.

The meaning you assign to your experiences will continually change your feelings; also, the quality of your life is gotten from the emotions you feel.

The meaning you assign to a situation can be wrong if seen through a distorted lens. As an example, a lack of trust will be the basis you assign to all future relationships if you were cheated on in a past relationship. This is only a side of the picture and cannot be categorized as either wrong or right.

Your happiness depends on you looking back at the events which have occurred and accepting what is and letting go of whatever you cannot control.

The way we think is what prevents us from attaining happiness, not luxury homes, a bank account full of money, or fancy cars. Although these things are good to have, they tend to wear out after a time and become meaningless if you are unable to feel contentment and peace on the inside.

Overthinking does not help you improve, neither does it allow you to experience the beauty in life. As a matter of fact, it is certain that you will begin to carry toxic emotions around.

Like stoic principles teach, worrying has no effect on events that have already occurred as they cannot be changed.

Accept and believe that whatever happened did so for your greater good instead of blaming yourself for what had happened.

Ways to Let Go of Past Hurts

Creating space for happiness and new joy in your life is the only way you can accept them. There is no way you can allow anything new to come into your heart if it is already filled up with hurt and pain.

1. Make the decision to let it go. Things do not just vanish on their own. You need to be committed to letting go of them. Self-sabotage can arise, preventing you from moving forward if you do not consciously decide to let the past hurt go.

You need to be able to understand that it is your choice to let it go when you consciously decide to do so. Stop thinking of the pain from the past. Stop reliving the memories, concerning the events in your head, every time you remember the other person (after you've gotten through with the second step below). This empowers most people as they become aware that they have the ability to either continue to feel the pain or live a life free from the pain.

2. Express your pain and responsibility. Give voice to the pain you felt from the hurt, either directly to the other person involved, or through removing it from your system (by writing in a journal, pouring it out to a friend, or even writing it down in a letter you will never deliver to the other person involved). Make sure you get it out of your system. This will help you know exactly what caused you to feel hurt.

We live in a world of gray, although it sometimes feels like we live in a world of white and black. However, the amount of responsibility from the pain you felt may not be the same, you might be partially responsible for it. What other option or step can you have undertaken? Were you actively participating in your own life or were you merely a victim? Will you allow your pain define who you are? Or will you become someone more complex and with more depth than that?

3. Stop playing the victim. Although, it feels good to be a victim, similar to belonging to a winning team against every other person. But you know what? The world just does not care, so you need to think again. True, you are unique. True, your feelings count. But do not mistake "your feelings count" for "your feelings above all things and no other thing matters." This thing called life is a whole lot of things like complex, messy, and interwoven and your emotions are merely a part of it.

In all steps of your life, you have a choice to either continue to allow the actions of another person's cause you to feel good or bad. Why will you allow someone who has hurt you in the past continue to have the power to hurt you in the present?

The problems in a relationship cannot be fixed by continuing to ruminate or overanalyze it. Never. Not in this world's entire history. Why then will you choose to think and spend a lot of energy on the person you felt hurt you?

4. Focus on the present — the here and now — and joy. It is now time to let go. Stop thinking about your past and let it go. Stop portraying a picture where you are the protagonist and always the victim of the other person's hurtful actions. You cannot change what has happened in the past, you can only ensure that today will be the best day of your life.

When you focus on the present, you do not have time to think of the past. Whenever you remember past events (as will happen once in a while), allow it only for a brief period of time. Then call yourself back into the present gently. Most people are able to do this with the help of a conscious signal, like telling themselves "it is alright. That happened in the past and I am now concentrating on my happiness."

Do not forget that there will be no space for positive things if we continue to fill our lives and brains with hurt feelings. You will have to choose to either continue to feel the pain or allow joy into your life.

5. Forgive them and yourself. Essentially everyone is entitled to our forgiveness, although we may be unable to forget their bad behaviors. Most times, we are unable to move past our stubbornness and pain and are unable to imagine granting forgiveness. Forgiveness does not mean "I concur with what you have done," instead it means "I forgive you despite not agreeing to your actions."

Forgiveness does not mean being weak. It actually portrays "I am a good individual, you are also a good individual, your actions have caused me pain but I wish to go on with my life and allow joy into it and I cannot do that until I let go of this."

Forgiveness is a method of letting go of something in a tangible manner. It is also a means of feeling empathy for the other person and attempting to put yourself in the other person's shoes.

How will you live with yourself in future happiness and peace, if you are unable to forgive yourself?

The key to enjoying happiness and stopping overthinking is acceptance.

Chapter 21: Give Your Best and Forget the Rest.

It is quite typical for you to feel inadequate to be able to manage certain cases when the need arises. It is human to fret over your ability to really deal with the issue appropriately. You may say you do not have enough money, or resources, or enough grit, not enough commitment, not enough strength, or brains for it.

Sometimes, everything seems to be happening all at once and you can't seem to keep up and you lapse into another bout of overthinking which ironically will only make the situation worse rather than help you manage it, notwithstanding the fact that you may even be prepared for it. Overthinking wears us out because of all the expectations we place on ourselves and the continuous need for perfection.

Have you ever considered that just putting in your best is ample and you don't have to fret over the things beyond your control? It's alright to be different, to be peculiar. It doesn't have to look like another person's life. You are allowed to have a completely different tale to tell.

Be more concerned about rendering your best endeavor instead of fretting over what the aftermath may be. In the face of some situations, the things that are out of your hands may very well be the determining factors of the end result. For this reason, fretting will do nothing for you, so just give the best you have to offer and leave everything to rest.

I guarantee you, you don't have to do anything extra, your best is your best and it will always pay handsomely one way or another. Endeavor to give your very best because, just think about it, your best is everything you can do concerning that issue. For some advice on how to keep on giving your best for better effectiveness :

- **Pour so much love on yourself.** Loving yourself is honestly the crux of life itself. From that deep-seated well of love for yourself, the inspiration to put in your best no matter what can truly arise. You become kinder, more benevolent, affectionate, driven, and every other trait you have always wished upon yourself when you begin to love yourself.

- **Stop with all the fault finding and idealism.** It is good to set high standards for ourselves until we start to fall into depression because they turn out to be unattainable. I know they say shoot for the stars and if you fall at least you will fall among the clouds but don't shoot yourself in the leg over it. Set a goal, put in your best efforts but don't beat yourself about it not turning out exactly how you want. Trust the process and have faith in the universe. No, the universe doesn't have it out for you!

- **Be conscious of your surroundings.** The best way to be the best you can do is to be attentive and conscious of the things going on around you. Also, beware of your reactions to every occurrence.

Consider your next actions, if it is what you should be doing and if it will profit you in the long run. Ask yourself if what you are doing at this very moment will help you to where you want to be in life. You don't need a life coach when you can answer these questions daily.

- **Be put together but also be fluid.** Like earlier mentioned, clarify your desires and your needs and specify what brings you joy. Certainty aids fluidity in life. Be sure not to overthink it, let it flow.

- **Don't forget that life is a process.** Don't try to hurry through life. You will get to your destination, just appreciate the process, including the trials and the wins. Live in the present and appreciate every moment and every breath you take.

- **Don't overthink it.** Let go of the fear of failing when you have left the rest. Negative thoughts stay longer and are painful. It will only cause you to overthink past events and the unknown future. More than anything, you know that most of the stories you weave in your head are false and baseless. Let them go!

- I'm not saying it will be easy to clear your head all the time but don't ever let negativity fester in your mind. You can choose not to react the way it wants you to, by slowly but surely letting it move over you. Yes, you can choose to be unaffected by those thoughts. Let them go! When you are finding it hard to erase them, weave a factual story in your head to replace the fallacies that negativity comes up with.

- **Stop being judgmental.** When you have something to say about basically everything that happens around you, you get the unwelcome opportunity to overanalyze and overthink things. Cut down on your opinion dishing and being judgmental. This helps you to truly leave the rest when you have done your best. You don't have to form an opinion on that incident that is really none of your business, or that person. You will be expending useful mental energy and only wearing yourself out. You get to give some breathing space to your brain when you ignore the temptation to opine or judge trivial things.

It Doesn't Have To Be Difficult.

People tend to think that if something is not difficult or hurting, then it is not the real deal. Everything can be easy depending on how we see it or go about it. Allow nature to mold and shape you. Submit yourself to change and love. Permit yourself to be loved wholly and take back your life from the clutches of fear.

Learn how to love. Thoroughly study it. Dedicate time to understand it. Let love find you, groom you, and mold you into a person who has never known pieces, into someone whose only memory is one of wholeness. This is why you live and breathe. This is the crux of life; love. Every other thing is just an addition. Believe in yourself and be inquisitive. Take charge of your life wholly!

Don't rush it, take your time. Win some, lose some, rise, fall, but rise again...and don't forget to laugh hard, and cry hard too. Sing, make music with your heart. Harmonize with the melodies of those who can hear your song. Be all this with faith and grace.

There's so much to do and think about, just do what you can do and leave the rest.

Chapter 22: Don't put Pressure on Yourself to Handle it.

Without knowing, many of us put additional stress on ourselves when we already encounter stress daily.

Excess pressure, accumulated with time, will most times cause a detonation. Of course, you won't actually detonate but you will have an emotional meltdown, an explosive fight with someone dear to you, or you become depressed when you are under self-imposed pressure or societal pressure.

Avoid putting yourself under excess pressure if you want to prevent physical and psychological dilemma. Even if the talk is cheap, you can be determined to let go of some situations. Be aware that you cannot transform suddenly but, with knowing yourself well, you can learn to try not to always be perfect.

Knowing when you are the cause of unneeded pressure is the first move for reducing the pressure on yourself. Don't beat yourself up for this general behavior, rather find out things to do to quit wrecking yourself and become your most powerful partner in removing stress.

Now, how can we find and free pressure points? I demand you to:

- Pinpoint your "pressure points". Questions like,

"How have I been placing pressure on myself in different aspects of my life(my love life specifically)?" will help a great deal.

- Also ask this, What is the effect of my pressure points on my interactions with people and my life as a whole?

- Now attempt to pinpoint the origin of the pressure points. The question, Where is this pressure from? Be thorough and frankly true to yourself.

These are a few best methods to maximize your life and reduce self-given stress as a result of overthinking

Make mistakes, it's okay. Even if no one likes mistakes, it is frequently bound to happen. How else are we supposed to learn?

Quit giving yourself impractical principles. Everyone makes mistakes and these mistakes shape us into the people we are at the moment.

Don't be scared of disgracing yourself or spoiling things. Without mistakes, we will not know the things that are suitable for us and those that aren't. Strangely, mistakes are eventually positive.

Grab opportunities, commit errors, mess things up. When you eventually move beyond flinching, the ordeal and the knowledge gained will make you glad.

Think like an optimistic realist rather than a pessimist. A lot of people are scared of thinking positively, they compare it to a mind game in which you disregard relevant issues or beneficial pointers that life gives and end up committing errors that will cause additional stress.

An optimistic method you can use is positive thinking, it is a set manner of thinking that allows you to concentrate on the achievements that increase your self-esteem and allow you to give your best in the future.

Stop comparing yourself to others. There is no other person like you. This should give you pleasure. Quit measuring yourself against other people, particularly regarding impractical standards. There is no other person like you nor like the fellow you are measuring yourself against.

Acknowledge who you are and show off! The fact that you do not resemble another person should not let you feel inferior. Consistently measuring yourself against others compels you to only concentrate on the unfavorable.

Be thankful for your special characteristics. It is specific to only you. Be thankful for how you've been treated. Concentrate on the awesome things about you. When you are capable of properly appreciating yourself, being optimistic becomes easy and you can do away with pessimistic thoughts that try to crawl into your mind.

One of the toughest things we can do is forgetting. But if you can forget the things that burden you, becoming optimistic in life is easily achieved. Carrying out these processes will aid in removing the pressure and allow you to live free and be happy.

Realize nothing is that important. Is it that PowerPoint presentation for your boss or preparing invitations for your first child's birthday? In the big plan, nothing is relevant enough to make you get exhausted, annoyed, or sad.

Nothing is worth losing your night's rest over. Don't get so worried that you become ill. Rather, inhale, exhale, then get answers to the questions stated beforehand. This will aid to put things in order.

Don't put too much pressure on yourself. Nothing should be taken too seriously.

Chapter 23: Journal to get the Thoughts out of your Head.

There are various reasons journaling is a highly recommended thinking management tool. Many types of research have shown the effectiveness of journaling for happiness, health, and stress management. It is a simple and enjoyable technique. There are different means of journaling with everyone standing a chance to benefit from it. The habit of journaling should be added to your life, you can journal daily, weekly, or as much as you need in case the stress becomes too intense.

One way journaling stops overthinking is by helping you go through your thoughts. This is because overthinking can cause rumination and mental stress if not controlled, although, some reasons for your overthinking can be reduced through a little focused examination. Journaling can be a great way of checking and moving thoughts from ruminative and anxious thoughts to action-oriented and empowering thoughts.

How to Get Started

You can get yourself out of an area of stress and be relieved in a few minutes by following the plan below. Are you ready? Get a pen or open a document and let's go!

Begin by journaling for 5 to 15 minutes. Write down your thoughts and those things disturbing you:

- Write down your worries and continue to do so until you feel you have put down the things needed to be said without going into rumination. You might wish to use a journal, computer, or even a paper and pen. If you make use of paper, endeavor to leave a line or two for every line used as this will be useful later on.

- Explain what is happening at that moment and the events presently causing difficulties. Do not forget that with overthinking, it is not always what is presently occurring that causes stress but your worries about what can happen in the future. If this is so for you, it is okay; you can put down what is occurring presently and indicate that the only part which is really stressful is what will occur next. (This can, in fact, lead to relief from stress itself).

- Next, write out your fears and worries and put it down in order of time from the earliest to the latest. This means that you start with one of the things causing you stress in the present and think about what it can lead to. Then put down your fears on what will occur afterward.

- Write out its effect on you.

Once your thoughts are in order, look for what you can do to reduce some of the anxiety and stress within.

Journaling Your Way to a Better Frame Of Mind

Putting your fears and concerns to paper goes a long way in removing those thoughts from your head and into the open. Next, read again and think through what you have written.

Examination of your cognitive distortion helps you see the benefit of changing the habit of stress-inducing thought patterns.

- Once you have observed what is of concern to you at present, look into your other options. Is it possible for there to be changes right now? Are there things you can do to change events or your thoughts on issues?

- When you write out what you fear will happen next,

think logically and endeavor to argue with yourself. Write out whatever comes into question if it is really a concern or not. How possible is it that this will occur and how you know it will occur? How sure are you? If your concerns really do occur, is it possible that it will not be as negative as you expected it to be? Is it possible that it becomes neutral or even better a positive event? Is it possible that you can use your circumstances to make a better result for yourself, making use of the things available to you and the possible changes that can occur? What better change can you bring?

You now understand. Facing your fears usually helps you relieve anxiety. You begin to see that things are unlikely to occur once you think that they are either bad or not as bad as you believe they can be.

- For every concern or fear you have, endeavor to write out at least one or two ways which you can see it in a different manner. Create a brand-new story for yourself, a new set of potential occurrences, and put it down on paper beside your fears which you are thinking about.

- Examination of your cognitive distortion can also help you see the benefit of changing the habit of stress-inducing thought patterns.

It can be quite helpful to process what you feel on paper. Write it out, prepare for the worst, and hope for the best.

Chapter 24: Change the Channel.

Never let yourself get bored with life, always keep yourself busy with anything that interests you. Take part in any activity that excites you and can also take your mind off worries. We all face different challenges in life but we should not concentrate on them. However, an idle mind has no choice but to worry and overthink about the issues surrounding life. The less busy you are, the more time you have to worry. Therefore, it is very necessary that you get yourself any form of distraction, something that can indulge your mind and take off anxieties.

Notice that most of the time when you are engaging in anything that gives you joy, your mind seems to be free from thoughts but just soaking in the moment and this is when you can say "I had a good time". When you are busy living every second of your life by doing this (getting involved with every activity that excites you); you tend to forget about your worries, thereby relieving your mind of stress.

Distract yourself with activities like sports, planting, seeing a movie, even conversation with loved ones. Whatever you choose to distract yourself with must be something you love and is able to draw your attention away from anxieties. Your distraction must also be something that can be done on a regular basis. If you have a lot of hours to spare, you can even consider offering voluntary service to children, the elderly, even animals. Being of help to other people is another way to distract yourself from your own problems and concentrate on others. It also helps you to feel useful, instead of worrying about things you don't have control over.

Finding a distraction is like trying to heal a broken heart. It is a way of helping you to move on from the pain and hurt, it helps you to reconsider facts and appreciate life more. Distractions are like good friends who constantly help us to find ourselves when we are lost.

This skill (distraction skill) is often used in the medical field to calm patients and distract them from pain or any other form of uneasiness. This is to show that this skill or art is very necessary for all fields of life. The aim of distracting ourselves is to give us the opportunity to experience other things that we can be grateful for. It opens our eyes to see the world around us and to appreciate it.

Once you begin to get yourself more involved with life, not creating any space for anxious feelings and worries, you will notice the positive mindset that comes with peace of mind.

There are endless lists of distractions you can engage in, but a few are listed below;

- The habit of listening to relaxing music
- Get a pet you can snuggle with
- Taking tea or having your best snack
- Opt-in for long walks
- Exercise

- Be engaged in sports
- Read a book
- You can write
- Lay still for a while or take a nap
- Clean the house
- Go out shopping, meeting friends, or just go strolling
- Draw
- Recite rhymes or ABCs

Whatever you do, just get a hobby. Distract yourself to get out of the loop

Chapter 25: Take A Break.

You can be dragged down by problems when you are simply trying to concentrate on the present job or you just want to have fun.

When experiencing a situation that is beyond your control, searching for a positive activity to engage in is a healthy option. Search for a distraction, something that brings pleasure or comfort, or makes you feel better.

Relaxing in nature is refreshing, calming, and a great reliever of stress and worry. Any time you find yourself overburdened by thoughts running rampant in your mind, step out for a walk down the beach, by the river, or in the park.

The aim is to connect with yourself. Concentrate on the sounds, sights, and smells of your surroundings. Going on a break will take your mind away from your worries, make you calm, and comfort you.

Break for Results

Creating time for physically and mentally refreshing breaks is easy. Search for an activity that you enjoy. Select from these options to try out during your next break.

Stretching. If you are like a lot of people that sit at a computer or a desk for a long time, stand up from your chair at least once every hour to move around and stretch your legs and arms. Additionally, regularly taking your eyes away from the screen makes your eyes less tired.

Walking. Walking movements speed up circulation, causing you to be more active and reducing the tension in your muscles. Additionally, a change in environment might give you a new solution or viewpoint to a lingering problem.

Breathing. Inhaling slow, deep breaths through the nose and exhaling from the mouth is a form of exercise to control breathing. This is a great method of refreshing your mind, relieving tension, and improving alertness. You can practice these breathing exercises by lying down or sitting in a chair. For effective results, try doing up to 8 repetitions twice or thrice in a day.

Exercise. Whenever you can, take that bicycle ride or that 20-minute walk. Short periods of exercise increase your heart rate and improve circulation, make you more alert, keep your weight under control, improve your appetite, and make you less tired.

Visualization. One strategy to obtain the positive effects of a serene environment when you cannot be present there, in reality, is by Visualization. For example, if you are having a rough day at work, you can lie down or sit in a chair for some minutes and imagine being in a favorite vacation spot or sitting in a comforting hot tub that is causing all the stress to melt away. Visualize as many exciting details as you can: smells, sounds, and sights. This transmits impulses to your brain, telling it to slow down.

Read a book. A little distraction is all that is needed to escape from the confinement. Forget about the Internet and read a book. Become engrossed in a romantic story or read something that takes you to a different place and time. If it is impossible to take away your worries, take yourself away from them.

Help someone else. Stop being selfish. Think about other people. Become a local volunteer, donate to a good cause, make sandwiches for the homeless people in your area. The easiest way to stop thinking about yourself is to think about another person.

A lot of those things that will weigh us down and make us lose sleep can be fixed by some hours of enjoyment, pleasure, or distraction, instead of another stressful day filled with worry and anxiety.

When adopting these strategies, follow the directions of your body and do not allow strict routine to dictate your breaks. When your breaks become relegated to another duty on your to-do list, it will be hard to get your desired benefits. So, take that break when you desire it most.

Your mood, alongside your perspective, will be improved. Everything, including the impossible challenges in life, appears to be easier when you take a break from all the stress. A little breathing room can preserve your perspective and help you explore other options for a positive change.

Consolidate all your problems instead of leaving

them to interrupt your daily life.

Chapter 26: Work out.

Your health, as well as your daily activities, can be negatively impacted by overthinking. Like you know already, the process of overthinking is tedious, it takes up a greater part of your time and prevents you from engaging in profitable activities.

You tend to regard every situation as too complex and your brain becomes stressed from overanalyzing. So it is very difficult to deploy your problem-solving and analytical skills. Most times, you are upset and disappointed with yourself. Eventually, these result in anxiety and depression. Little things start to terrify you or irritate you, you might even cry. In addition, there is a speedup in the process of aging, there is a shift in your sleep pattern, and you might experience an eating disorder.

Not only does working out help to limit overthinking but it also reduces the internal stress and anxiety.

Like we know, there is no way you can switch off your brain if you do not want to think. The process is hard, but it is harmless to try and you can also enhance the quality of your life while doing this.

You need a great deal of mental concentration to engage in an intense workout, this implies that all your concentration will be on the exercise, instead of the several imaginations running through your mind.

Also, endorphins are released in your brain when you work

out, leading to a general feeling of wellness and positivity. This reduces the risk of thinking disturbing or negative thoughts.

How Exercise Promotes Positive Well-Being

People who feel mentally healthy can also improve their health by exercising. Engaging in physical activity has been discovered to stimulate quality sleep, improve moods, and boost energy levels.

The benefits of physical activity for mental health are numerous, they include:

Stress hormones are reduced by exercising. Stress hormones, such as cortisol, are reduced when you work out. Endorphins- your positivity hormone- are also released when you work out and this helps to improve your mood.

Physical activity deflects your attention from negative emotions and thoughts. Physical activity distracts you from your problem, channels your mind to your present activity or move you into a calm state.

Exercise increases confidence. Working out helps to tone your muscles, lose weight, and achieve a healthy smile and radiance. You might experience a slight but significant improvement in your mood, your clothes fit better, and you emanate an aura of renewed confidence.

Exercise can be an excellent source of social support. There are proven benefits of social support and a lot of physical activities can be regarded as social activities too. Thus, it does not matter whether you play softball in a league or become a member of an exercise class, group workout can give the added benefits of relieving stress.

Improved physical health equals improved mental health. Although stress results in illness, illness can result in stress as well. Enhancing your general wellness and longevity by exercising can prevent a lot of stress short-term, by increasing your immunity to the flu, colds, and other minor illnesses. And long-term by improving your health for a long while, helping you get the best out of life.

Exercise shields you from stress. There might be a link between physical activity and reduced physiologic response to stress. In simpler terms, stress has a reduced effect on people who actively workout. In addition to other benefits, exercise might make you immune to potential stress and can help you manage stress presently.

Types of Exercises to Overcome Overthinking

These three exercises that will assist you to defeat the practice of overanalyzing and overthinking. Stick to this incredible pattern and turn your life around.

Experiment with yoga. A great way to reduce the pressure on your brain and relieve stress is by practicing yoga. Yoga helps to channel your attention and concentration from insignificant things to your breathing and body by entering into a state of meditation.

Experiment with the Easy Pose in Yoga. Contrary to what the name implies, it is not easy. You sit with your hip bones flattened to the floor and extend your spine. Relax your shoulders and loosen your face to a state of tranquility. Drop your arms onto your knees and take deep breaths for at least one minute. This will get rid of all your worry and mental stress.

'Knees to Chest' is one other great exercise. The only thing you are required to do is lie back and hug your knees close to your chest. Make rocking movement sideways and take deep breaths for a minimum of 40 seconds.

Routine cardiovascular exercises. This is one great method of relaxation. Endorphins are natural pain relievers that are released during prolonged periods of increased heart rate. Not only does regular exercise decrease the level of stress in your body but it can also help with weight loss, increasing your confidence. If you are a newbie, try out these relatively simple exercises.

Begin by taking a walk on the hills. You can include ankle weights or use wrist straps or dumbbells to increase your heart rate. Otherwise, use a treadmill; turn on your preferred choice of music to prevent your brain from being distracted to insignificant things. Cycling is another great option if you do not enjoy walking.

Using the stairs is another option. Run or walk on the stairs, two at a time for about 10-15 seconds, otherwise, experiment with the Stairmaster at the gym.

Engage in Progressive muscle relaxation. This is a two-stage process. Firstly, you contract then relax various muscles in your body. This helps to neutralize the stress and tense muscles in your body. A relaxed body equals a relaxed mind. Keep in mind to ask your doctor about any history of back or muscle pain before doing this so that you can avoid the exacerbation of an underlying injury.

You can begin with your right foot. Tightly squeeze for 10 seconds, then allow it to relax. Do this also with your left foot and ascend in the same manner. Remember to take deep and slow breaths throughout.

Stress is decreased by engaging in routine physical activity

Chapter 27: Get a Hobby.

Doing something we love gives us happiness and makes our lives improved. This is a good method of quitting your overthinking habit. Have a constant artistic escape you love. Anything productive like programming, graphics designing, music, drawing and painting, being involved in a sport, and others.

The greatest method of starting another hobby is to attempt something different. There are awesome and fun activities worldwide that we can delve into and convert to ours. It provides something interesting to do while we are free and gives the freedom to obtain additional skills. Your hobby can be playing video games.

We are all specific and different, hence, our hobbies and passions differ. And immediately we get a hobby we love and that truly interests us, we are glued to it. It develops into an integral aspect of our lives and fascinates us personally. If your thoughts should become overwhelming, carry out your hobby and get engrossed in it. Stick to it till you feel revitalized.

There are numerous reasons why we all should pick up a hobby but these are some major benefits:

- **It makes you more interesting.** Having hobbies opens you to diverse encounters, so you will have loads of stories to tell. They are specialists in that area so they can lecture anyone that is curious about their topics.

- **It helps to relieve stress by keeping you engaged in something you enjoy.** Hobbies are outlets to escape the stress of daily living. They allow you to rest and find joy in exercises that are not work-related or related to other obligations.

- **Hobbies help you become more patient.** To acquire a new hobby, you have to be calm to learn to do something you've never done before. Chances are, there will be a learning period and patience will be required to hone your skills.

- **Having a hobby can help your social life and create a bond with others.** A hobby is an activity you constantly take pleasure in with others. If you are part of a club, participate in a league, or just help others with the outcome of your work, a hobby is an awesome avenue to meet and bond with people that are passionate about the same things you are passionate about.

- **It helps you develop new skills:** Dedicating and giving your time to a hobby, leads to you building new skills. You continue to be better at a hobby as the time you spend at it increases.

- **It helps prevent bad habits and wasting time:** The saying "idle hands are the devil's workshop" never gets old. Having good hobbies to do during your free time ensures that you do not spend that free time on negative or wasteful activities.

- **It increases your confidence and self-esteem:** The odds are that enjoying an activity usually guarantees that you will be good at it. Excelling in any activity helps you develop pride in your accomplishments and build up your confidence.

- **It increases your knowledge:** Developing your hobby not only guarantees to build new skills but it also ensures you gain new knowledge.

- **It challenges you:** In partaking in a new hobby, you begin to engage in activities which are new and challenging. If it is not challenging for you, your hobby will be less enjoyable and you may not find it engaging.

- **Hobbies help reduce or eradicate boredom:** Hobbies ensures that you have something to do in your free time. They also ensure that you have something to be excited about and something to look forward to.

- **It enriches your life and gives you a different perspective on things:** It is certain that you will have access to new ideas no matter the hobby you choose. Hobbies also assist you by helping you to grow in several ways including giving you new ways to see life and giving you new opinions.

Your focus is shifted from overthinking into the present activity when you become involved in your hobby. This helps to show your creativity and enhances your coordination and cognitive function.

Chapter 28: Don't Be Too Hard On Yourself.

Oftentimes, you overthink as a result of being very tough on yourself. Your desire for fortune is so much that you wallow in anguish if your plans do not come through. You are still angry at yourself for your recent failure.

Since we all desire a better tomorrow, we tend to be bothered and think too much about how our tomorrow will be. You are bothered about losing your employment, about your company drowning, that a divorce is imminent, and many other things.

Stop it! Because being bothered will not change anything.

In a real sense, it ruins your present moment. Accept the fact that you cannot do anything about your tomorrow and stop bothering yourself about it.

If you are often being too tough on yourself, eliminating your overthinking behavior becomes a problem. In reality, life never goes as planned.

At times, things will not turn out well and there's nothing wrong with that. Prepare to let go of the guilt when things do not turn out as planned. Often, you are not the cause.

Why bother over a situation you cannot do anything about?

Immediately when you desist from being tough on

yourself, failure will not elicit fear in you, leading to less overthinking.

Acknowledge that your tomorrow will come to pass as it was meant to and direct your strength to activities that will give you pleasure and satisfaction.

How to Stop Being Too Hard on Yourself

It is crucial to be tolerable and appreciate yourself to end being tough on yourself. Instead of squandering time on self-guilt, teach yourself to make living better for you.

- **Have realistic expectations.** You are only human, so understand that there's nothing wrong with making errors. There is no flawless person and life is not flawless. Making errors will help you gain knowledge and develop, and how you want life is not often what you get. Accept your life's course, be dedicated to acquiring knowledge and getting better as a person. Concentrate only on things you can actually influence.

- **Look for the lessons in everything.** Rather than punishing yourself when a mistake is made, accept the wrong and search for the morals in it. It is okay to be criticized but make sure the critics are useful and have relative importance. Having low self-confidence is closely associated with being overly tough on yourself. Be determined to not be tough on yourself. Question yourself on what you can do better in the future based on what you learned. See these encounters as a room for progress.

- **Challenge your negative inner critic.** The things you say and think about are important and being pessimistic will disfigure your existence. Repetitively questioning yourself will add nothing to you. Layoff living on your errors. This is a misuse of strength, it is unhelpful and keeps you stagnated. Fight the pessimism and concentrate on progress.

- **Focus on the positives.** There is "good" everywhere but you will most likely not notice them if you are tough on yourself. Deliberately look for the positives. Question yourself on the things you did correctly, what you appreciate about you and your existence. Getting a journal and writing it out is helpful.

- **Put things in perspective.** Are the errors you committed and your life as tragic as you imagine it to be? In about 10 years, will it still be important? You can talk to a reliable person about it.

- **Use affirmations.** For instance "I might not be the best but I'm obtaining knowledge and progressing" or "what I did then was to the best of my knowledge."

- **Treat yourself as a best friend.** Accept yourself as someone with flaws, treat yourself with tenderness, and shower yourself with love. Allow yourself to do new things, commit errors, figure things out, and make progress. Cherish yourself and know your complete value.

Progress is halted when you are too tough on yourself. But you can stop being tough on yourself. It requires determination and strength, but it is worthwhile. If you have any issue or you think you're always stagnated, feel free to ask for assistance. Desist from being tough on yourself, cultivate self-confidence, and build the kind of life you desire.

You do not have to be in charge. Accept that you can do nothing about tomorrow and you have no power over everything.

Quit being an idealist

Chapter 29: Get Plenty of Good Quality Sleep.

In maintaining a beneficial attitude and not getting carried away with an adverse mentality, sleep is a majorly forgotten factor. When you do not get adequate sleep, you are prone to get bothered and have negative thoughts, you do not meditate with your usual clarity, and you get carried away with the various thoughts whirling in your mind while you overthink.

To gain and retain knowledge, to be innovative, a bright and attentive brain is required. Conversely, more errors are made and there is a reduction in creativity in our activities when you do not get enough sleep.

Adequate sleep ensures that we have the right mental state to obtain information in our daily activities. Also, adequate sleep is required to refine and memorize that information over a long period of time. Sleep causes alterations in the brain which consolidates the thought- reinforcing network amongst brain cells and sending information through the hemispheres of the brain.

Benefits of Sleeping

- **Sharpens your attention.** You will have observed that it is hard to focus on things when you have too many thoughts whirling in your head. It is difficult to learn a lot of new things when you overthink. If you are properly relaxed, you will have more clarity and an acute focus.

- **Sleep boosts your mental health.** Go to bed timely for your intellectual health. Sleep reduces signs of depression. Lack of sleep can cause anxiety and increase stress. When you are too tense to sleep, you can leave your bed, try to meditate, or write in a journal to aid in setting your mind for sleep.

- **Improves your memory.** Making a memory is three phases. Phase one is acquisition, this is where you bring facts into your mind. Phase two is consolidation; here, the information is solidified. Lastly, recall - and it's just what you think, we can go back to the saved information. Phases one and three occur during our wakeful hours and phase two occurs during our sleeping hours. During sleep, the brain consolidates and arranges our thoughts, this aids in recalling previously acquired knowledge.

- **Lowers your stress.** When you don't get enough sleep, have you observed how unimportant things get you worried? Too much thinking causes you to be surly and have adverse reactions to insignificant inconveniences and interference. Sleep aids in decreasing stress.

- **It helps decision making.** Your sleep affects your decisions. Having a time of inert thinking, like sleep, aids good decision making. Do you know anyone that wants to make a life-changing decision tired?

- **It helps you focus on your tasks.** If you are not sleeping well for yourself, sleep well for your duties. Research tells us that sleep will help you stay conscious and attentive all through the day, allowing your schedule to work more than it will be if you did not sleep. Short naps can also sharpen your concentration. Acquiring knowledge and tactical skills are made better by sleep.

- **Sleep physically clears your mind.** Just as you clear away garbage in your home, let sleep take out the garbage in your head. Toxins that gather over a period of time are cleaned by the brain when you sleep. That's probably why you feel very good when you get up from a great sleep.

How to Get The Most From Your Sleep

- **Learn how long you take to fall asleep.** If you want to sleep for a definite period of time, you actually have to consider the amount of time you use to fall asleep. A sleep-tracking mobile application can help with this. Once you've estimated this, consider it when thinking of your sleeping time.

- **Keep it cool.** Walking into a cozy bedroom is okay initially. However, I realized that I sleep more comfortably, peacefully, and with fewer nightmares in a cold room.

- **Keep the earplugs nearby.** If you are like me, you wake up at the slightest noise, then plain earplugs are the best thing. These low-cost materials have aided my good night rest and helped me sleep, even if there are loud cats, snorers, and any other interruption.

- **Don't try to force yourself to go to sleep.** Don't get in bed and compel yourself to sleep, when you are not feeling sleepy. From experience, doing this leads to rolling around in my bed for more than an hour. The best thing to do in a situation like this is to ease off for about 20-30 minutes on the sofa, by reading or anything you find suiting. Doing this causes me to sleep a lot more quickly and eventually get adequate sleep.

- **Don't sleep too long.** What initially made me hate taking naps was sleeping for the incorrect amount of time. What is wrong with this is that it can cause you to have sleep laziness - the feeling of wooziness and being weaker than you were before you went to sleep.

  As blood flow and temperature of the brain is lower during sleep, waking up unexpectedly and an increased level of brain function is unsettling.

  Sleeping for more than 90 minutes is not useful because you will start another sleep cycle. Also, napping at the end of the day will comprise of excess slow-wave sleep.

  Restrict your snooze to 15 minutes. 30 minutes can cause sleep inertia, or slowing of the prefrontal cortex of the brain that is in charge of judgment. To reboot this takes about 30 minutes.

  The general agreement common to all the studies I researched is either to go for a 15-20 minute short nap, possibly drinking some coffee ahead of time, to get up with more energy (but I'll be awed if you can pull this off), or to nap for a complete 90 minute sleep cycle and be awake before the beginning of the next cycle.

- **Choose the right time of day.** Snoozing when your strength levels are habitually lowered can aid in preventing the feeling of the feared limitless hour when the day slowly continues as you fight your sleepiness. For those that work the usual 9-5, this time is normally post lunch: due to the innate cycle of our circadian rhythm, we are tired twice in 24 hours. The middle of the night is one of the heights of sleepiness and the other about 12 hours later is right in the mid-afternoon.

If you did not get adequate sleep the previous night, the plunge in thoughts will be felt more powerfully, so you will want to nap more. Instead of battling this feeling with coffee and energy drinks, you can nap shortly to freshen your brain before you face the afternoon.

- **Practice.** To improve napping, practice is important. Finding what is specific to you can take time, so keep trying various times of the day, various nap lengths, and various methods of waking.

  Ensure that your sleeping environment has little light. Have a blanket handy to keep you warm while sleeping.

Get adequate quality sleep. Keep it cool. Keep the earplugs close. Don't force yourself to go to sleep.

Conclusion.

You need to train yourself to stop overthinking and make a conscious effort to practice this daily for it to become a habit. Controlling your feelings and thoughts requires serious practice and commitment.

On its own, your thoughts can drift randomly from one idea to another, it can go down memory lane, chase wild thoughts, or stir up bitter ideas or resentment and anger. Alternatively, your mind can dive into a sea of daydreaming and a world of fantasy, if care is not taken, your life can be controlled by such random thoughts such that every decision or action you take becomes unpredictable. Such intrusive thoughts you might experience during the day is evidence that most of the functions of the mind are likely beyond conscious control. In addition, our thoughts can feel so powerful and real and it can affect the way we perceive the outside world.

Take a moment to discard the assumption that your spontaneous thoughts are meaningless and totally harmless. In truth, such thoughts may be meaningless at that moment, they can be the product of past memory or emotion but in the present moment, they might not reflect reality.

Most of our thoughts are under the control of our subconscious mind and our subconscious mind will never grant us total control over our thoughts. However, you still have the capacity to control some of your thoughts. Also, you can change some of your habits and how you react to them to gain more control over your emotions.

As you went through this book, you have found a various selection of ideas and tools that can help you to declutter your mind so that you can mute all the negative voices in your head, reduce stress, and have more peace of mind.

Making conscious efforts to avoid overthinking is a rewarding course of action which will impact the quality of your life significantly. By spending less time going through intrusive, negative thoughts "in your mind" you will have more time to enjoy the present moment and every other moment.

References

7 Reasons Productive People Go to Bed Early. (2019). Retrieved from https://www.inc.com/amy-morin/7-reasons-productive-people-go-to-bed-early.html

Michl, L., McLaughlin, K., Shepherd, K., & Nolen-Hoeksema, S. (2013). Rumination as a mechanism linking stressful life events to symptoms of depression and anxiety: Longitudinal evidence in early adolescents and adults. *Journal Of Abnormal Psychology*, *122*(2), 339-352. doi: 10.1037/a0031994

Nolen-Hoeksema, S., Wisco, B., & Lyubomirsky, S. (2008). Rethinking Rumination. *Perspectives On Psychological Science*, *3*(5), 400-424. doi: 10.1111/j.1745-6924.2008.00088.x

Thomsen, D., Yung Mehlsen, M., Christensen, S., & Zachariae, R. (2003). Rumination—relationship with negative mood and sleep quality. *Personality And Individual Differences*, *34*(7), 1293-1301. doi: 10.1016/s0191-8869(02)00120-4

www.ingramcontent.com/pod-product-compliance
Lightning Source LLC
Chambersburg PA
CBHW071712020426
42333CB00017B/2234